Praise for *Helping Your Children*

"Although my kids weren't born until after n
become really important for me
is an illness that affects the wh
cancer survivorship experience
Cancer provides valuable advice
on the whole family. The person
tance of opening a dialogue for c
gain the knowledge they need to

> — Lance Armstrong

"Helping your children cope with your cancer can be a way for you to show how much you care about and love them. It will be the hardest thing you have ever done and this book and the personal stories and programs contained in it will help you do it the best way for you and your child."

> — Peggy Anne Mur
> Les Gallo-Silver, ...S.W.R..
> and Stacy Kramer, L.M.S.W., *Cancer Care, Inc.*

"This book provides an instant support group for families in which a parent has been diagnosed with cancer. The book consists of 28 essays written by professionals, parents, and children. The essays written by parents give specific advice about how to help a child deal with a parent's cancer. The children's touching essays describe feelings of fear and regret of parent's illness."

> — *The Susan G. Komen Foundation*

"A remarkable publication, the first of its kind...essential to every family afflicted with cancer."

> — William R. Nelson, M.D.,
> *former Surgical Oncologist Fellow,*
> *Memorial Sloan-Kettering Center*

"This innovative book offers parents, teachers, mental health professionals, and caregivers practical tools with which to help children find a sense of security in this unexpected life experience."

— Linda Lister, Ph.D., *psychologist, author,*
and creator of the Great Girls program

"A special gift from families affected by cancer to families affected by cancer. A moving collage of very human stories that will let you laugh and cry—and give you hope and courage. Cancer affects all of us. These personal stories will help us confront cancer with more love, hope, and understanding."

— Mary Anne Mills, M.S.W.,
hospice social worker and Race for the Cure volunteer

"Helping Your Children Cope With Your Cancer...is a wonderful resource for people who want to avoid the isolation that often develops in families that are coping with this terrible disease....(an) inspiring and thoughtful book....I recommend this book to parents, therapists, doctors and teachers who want to be sensitized to the inner lives of their children."

— Sonya Rhodes, Ph.D.
Author and Family Therapist, New York City
Consultant, Jewish Board of Children and Family
Services

"This is wonderfully written and should be very helpful to families struggling with their diagnosis and its impact on their children."

—Richard D. Krugman, M.D.
Professor of Pediatrics and Dean, University of
Colorado School of Medicine

"What is evident in these very personal stories is that in the face of pain, uncertainty and loss, the sharing of emotions becomes a source of healing. For children, particularly, getting back on the path of normal development requires honest communication and a heart-open stance. Peter van Dernoot's book speaks powerfully to this."

— Martha Kendall Ryan, Psy. D.
Clinical psychologist and adjunct professor at the
University of Denver Graduate School of Professional
Psychology

"Helping Your Children Cope With Your Cancer is a vital resource for families facing the diagnosis of cancer....This exceptionally moving book fills a critical niche which has been largely ignored by the health-care system. The entire family is a victim of cancer....It is important that they know that they are not alone and that there is help. This vision of a support group for children with a parent diagnosed with cancer should become an essential part of cancer health care."

— Betty Layne, D.D.S., M.S.D.
Director, National Planning and Policy
Alliance for Lung Cancer Advocacy, Support,
and Education (ALCASE)

"Children are often the silent victims of their parent's cancer. What should they be told? How much will they understand? This book addresses these very important and often ignored issues. The authors are to be congratulated on a fine piece of work and, more importantly, on recognizing the need for this book. This book should be required reading for all oncology professionals."

— Carl G. Kardinal, M.D.
Director, Ochsner Cancer Institute
New Orleans, LA

HELPING your CHILDREN COPE with your CANCER

A GUIDE FOR PARENTS AND FAMILIES

SECOND EDITION

HELPING your CHILDREN COPE with your CANCER

A GUIDE FOR PARENTS AND FAMILIES
SECOND EDITION

Peter van Dernoot

With insights from parents, children, Madelyn Case, Ph.D., and Cancer Care, Inc.

HATHERLEIGH PRESS
NEW YORK • LONDON

Published by Hatherleigh Press
5-22 46th Avenue, Suite 200
Long Island CIty, NY 11101
Toll Free 1-800-528-2550
Visit our websites getfitnow.com and hatherleighpress.com

Hatherleigh Press books are available for bulk purchase, special promotions and premiums. For more information on reselling and special purchase opportunities, please call us at 1-800-528-2550 and ask for the Special Sales Manager.

Library of Congress Cataloging-in-Publication Data

Van Dernoot, Peter
  Helping your children cope with your cancer: with insights from parents, children, and Madelyn Case / Peter van Dernoot
    p. cm.
  Includes Index.
  ISBN-13: 978-1-57826-231-1
  ISBN-10: 1-57826-231-3
    Children of cancer patients 2. Cancer—Patients—Family relationships 3. Cancer—Psychological aspects I. Case, Madelyn. II. Title

RC262.V36 2002
362.1'96994—dc21   2001059395

Cover Design by Angel Harleycat
Interior Design and Layout by Fatema Tarzi

10 9 8 7 6 5 4 3 2 1
Printed in Canada on acid-free paper.

With love to my two great (grown) kids, Craig and Laura.

I wish I had done more.

The net proceeds from the sale of this book will be used principally to fund The Children's Treehouse Foundation, a national nonprofit organization the author has established to provide support for children whose parents have cancer. Visit www.childrenstreehousefdn.org.

Acknowledgments

This book could not have been compiled without the support of dozens of individuals and far too many organizations to name.

A few deserve special thanks, however, for their particular interest and help:

- Avon Foundation Breast Cancer Crusade

- The American Cancer Society for statistical data.

- The National Coalition for Cancer Survivorship for posting my project and request for letters on their Web site for several months.

- Gilda's Club, Inc. for informing its membership.

- The Alliance for Lung Cancer Advocacy, Support and Education for supporting the project in their newsletter.

- Oncology Nursing Society

- Cancer Care Inc.

- Susan G. Komen Foundation

- Memorial Sloan-Kettering Center　.

- *Colorado Parent*

- *People Weekly* magazine

- Sue Miller, founder of the Day of Caring, who inspired cancer survivors across the country to participate.

- Jeanne Currey, R.N., and Madelyn Case, Ph.D., Licensed Psychologist, the creators and guiding forces behind the Support Group for Children of Parents with Cancer at Porter Adventist Hospital in Denver, Colorado, and unflagging supporters of this project.

- Robin Martinez, a diligent "list owner" of the Association of Cancer On-line Resources, Inc. (ACOR, at <www.acor.org>), and Bonnie Sue McInturff, who was known to her many friends on the Internet as Bhost Bonz.

- Dr. Wendy S. Harpham, mother, wife, cancer survivor, and prolific writer on this subject, for her significant editorial input and encouragement of this book.

- The University of Colorado Health Sciences Center.

- My editor, Heather Ogilvie, for improving the flow and overall readability of this work.

- And many medical professionals and people who simply care... Dr. William R. Nelson; Dr. Lee Jennings; Dr. Michael Fenoglio; Jill Stoeffler, R.N.; Mary Anne Mills, M.S.W.; and my dear friend, Carol Sullivan, a cancer survivor herself and mother of two grown kids, who was the first person to know of this project concept and a wonderful inspiration throughout.

Virtually every cancer-related organization in the United States was invited to help provide letters for this book, as were a dozen of the country's leading cancer treatment centers. They all strongly endorsed the project, and most said they would help supply letters. So did scores of individual cancer survivors, including a major-league baseball player, a high school counselor, a medical doctor, a widow with two young children, and others.

Everyone praised the concept and underscored the need for such a collection of experiences. Said one authority, "The need is overwhelming. Much more needs to be written on the subject." Indeed, in the process, I've received a number of calls, letters, and e-mails asking for sources of information I may have discovered on helping kids cope with a parent's cancer.

And yet a strange phenomenon evolved: Although lauding the project objectives, most organizations and individuals found it difficult to follow through. As individuals sat down to put pen to paper, all too often it brought back such deep, painful memories that they were unable to record their thoughts. Some letter writers found themselves in tears as they wrote of their experiences.

I fully understand this. I've walked in those shoes, too. More than anything else, however, this simply emphasizes the essential need for appropriate communication with children who are living through a parental-cancer situation. If parents cannot express their thoughts months or years later, isn't it all the more critical that we find ways to communicate with our kids when the subject is timely?

So it is that I am particularly grateful for those parents, from New York to California, who contributed their very personal stories. Each one is a lesson in caring. Each has an important message. I am in their debt.

—*Peter R. van Dernoot*

Preface

Cancer is bad news—it's frightening even to think about.

According to the American Cancer Society and the U. S. Bureau of Census, approximately 315,247 parents, ages 25 to 54, will be diagnosed each year with invasive cancer. They then have the heart-wrenching task of breaking the frightening news to their more than 592,000 children under the age of 18.

Nothing compares to the emotional and psychological upheaval a family endures when a parent experiences cancer. Just ask any woman who, with sheer grit and determination, survives the disease only to have her marriage dissolve in the process. And if a parent is taken away, at any time—but especially when he or she hasn't seen the children grow into maturity—it is clearly one of life's great tragedies. In fact, psychologists say that among the many conflicting emotions that cancer-stricken mothers have is a feeling of failure—failure to be there to guide their children into adulthood.

If there is any good news, it is that scientists appear to be getting closer to identifying more clearly the causes of certain cancers and may be getting closer to their prevention.

Until then, families with this illness will continue to do the best they can, under extremely difficult emotional circumstances and with varying degrees of success.

Still, too little professional help and guidance is available to assuage or diminish the emotional trauma of the collateral casualties of parental cancer—the kids. In a sense, they are affected as greatly as their parents. Most assuredly, they will carry forever the memory and the emotional scars of their parent's illness, regardless of the outcome.

Sharing the experiences of how parents have eased that pain is the purpose of this book, and its origins lie with my own experiences.

These began when my wife was diagnosed with terminal cancer. My first reaction was absolute disbelief, as she had seemed the epitome of perfect health.

It was just as devastating for the kids. The news hit them like a lightning bolt.

Our son, 15-year-old Craig, bravely fought back the tears that welled up in his eyes. Laura, our 11-year-old daughter, exclaimed, "No!" and dissolved into tears.

My wife and I tried to soften it as much as possible. We avoided the technical terms that, prior to the previous two weeks, we'd never heard before: "stage four alveolar carcinoma of the lung." And we didn't use the word "terminal," principally because we didn't believe it ourselves.

But there it was. Our kids knew the implications.

We assured them that Mom was going to have more tests. We were going to do everything possible to fight this. We would talk with them openly about the illness so they would always know as much as we did. And they would always be loved and cared for.

There were a few things we didn't tell them. Since we'd received the diagnosis just five days before a planned Christmas ski vacation in Colorado, we asked the doctors if we should still take that trip, especially considering the cold and the higher altitude compared to our Chicago neighborhood.

They encouraged us to take the vacation trip with two bits of advice: Decide whether we wanted to get a second opinion at M. D. Anderson Cancer Center in Houston when we got back, and take the time to get our personal papers in order.

Accordingly, while in Denver, where we had lived for 16 years before taking a recent corporate job transfer to Chicago, we met with our lawyers to review and revise our legal documents before we headed up to the "hills" to ski.

We also had a heart-warming discussion with our best friends, at whose home we were spending the first two days. After dinner the first evening and after the kids had gone to bed, we told them about our situation. They were as devastated as we had been just a few days earlier. Not surprisingly, they asked, "Is there anything we can do?"

We had given this a lot of thought, given the critical nature of the diagnosis. Our immediate concern was the care and raising of our kids in the event my wife's diagnosis was correct, and in the unlikely circumstance that I got "hit by the proverbial bus."

"Would you consider being the godparents of our kids, taking them under your wing, should that be necessary?" I asked, adding they might want to think it over and give us an answer after we returned from the ski trip. To their wonderful credit, they said, "We don't have to think about it or wait a week. We love your kids and, of course, we will."

And, two days later, we called the doctor in Chicago and asked him to set up the appointment at M.D. Anderson.

We had decided not to dampen the enjoyment of the ski vacation by breaking the medical news to our kids. Instead, we opted to break the news after a lunch break on the long drive back to Chicago. This had allowed us adequate time to think through what we wanted to say and how we wanted to say it. Even so, given a secluded restaurant table away from the crowd and waitstaff dispatched, it was the hardest discussion we ever had with our children.

It was the beginning of an ongoing dialogue, extended by the tedium of Interstate 80's unswervingly direct passage through Nebraska in route to Chicago. (Laura had earlier proclaimed, "Dad, there's nothing out there but straight ahead!") With no potential interruptions, we were able to listen intently to their follow-up questions and concerns, and answer them as candidly and thoughtfully as we could. It was the beginning of an essential process.

During the two and a half years following that initial discussion and leading up to their mother's death, the kids each went through their own stages of denial, disbelief, anger, tolerance, and, finally, acceptance and helpfulness. And there were support groups: family, adult friends, the church, even the school varsity swim team, and more. Throughout the ordeal, as the kids moved on with their lives in the early years after her death, I thought they had weathered the storm satisfactorily. By his second year at college, Craig was enjoying life again and maturing well; Laura had a number of very close high-school friends and an active social life.

It is only from this perspective in time, nearly 20 years later, that I'm convinced that more should have been done to ease my children's pain. It is now evident to me: the pain and hurt of that type of ordeal may decrease over time, but it stays with the children for the rest of their lives.

When my wife was diagnosed with terminal cancer in 1980, no one suggested (or even knew of) programs to help our kids cope with their mom's cancer. Although a few resources now exist, such as the Internet, in general this issue is woefully ignored.

Recently, I discovered an organization uniquely qualified to help families manage this type of crisis. While on a public relations consulting assignment with Centura Health in Denver, I was introduced to a program developed by two visionary professionals at Centura's Porter Adventist Hospital. In 1993, while medical experts worked principally with the hospital's breast cancer patients, the support professionals became aware that something needed to be done to "stabilize" the emotions of their patients' children.

They began exploring possibilities: What should be done? What ages of children are we thinking about? What are their individual needs? Who can address them? Where will we get the funding and the time?

Within months, the Support Group for Children of Parents with Cancer was launched. This entirely free program, available to all families in the area, now has served dozens of kids ages 6 to 16, helping them to cope successfully with the trauma of a parent's cancer. (The program is now called Kids Alive!—Support for Children of Parents with Cancer.)

The fears and doubts that become pervasive, even debilitating, in young children, will evolve regardless of the parent's station in life. It is of no consequence that the parent is a national baseball star or well-known television celebrity, social worker or cab driver. The children, given the chance, will all show their pain and fear with the same questions and comments: "Is it my fault?" "Will Mom/Dad die?" "Will I get cancer?" "Where will we live?"

As I worked with the new support group, two thoughts emerged. First, more should have been done to ease the pain my own kids had experienced. And, second, it wasn't too late to do something to help other parents and kids who would find themselves in the same situation.

Over a period of many months, I have elicited personal stories from parents coast-to-coast on how they dealt with their cancer and, particularly, how they helped their kids cope with parental cancer.

This book has a narrow focus: Real-life stories of how some parents deal with their cancer and with the fears and anxieties of their children. The book won't go into the equally genuine pain felt by many others afflicted with or affected by cancer. Rather, it deals with the parent who has cancer and the collateral casualties: their children.

In each case, the cancer survivor or surviving spouse has written a short narrative on how a cancer affected them, the overall impact it had on their young children, and how they helped them cope. Wherever possible, I also asked the children (in some cases now young adults) to write their thoughts as well. I have been scrupulously faithful to their writings, editing only for clarity. These are their stories, and I am most appreciative.

Although each personal story is unique, a number of recurring themes have surfaced, pointing to the following advice:

- Provide honest, timely, open, ongoing conversation—it can help your children develop healthy, adaptive behavior with respect to your cancer. From the beginning, finding the right words in the right way (and even the courage to speak) is a defining step.

- Make the underlying message to your children that you're doing everything possible to win the cancer battle, and that your love and caring of them continues unabated.

- Encourage and enable your children to express their thoughts and concerns. Young children may choose to make drawings; older children may wish to write. Keep a journal for discussion.

- Expect to repeat elements of your discussion with your children. Just as adults do not satisfactorily process information in a crisis, children need to hear explanations more than once.

- Understand that cancer affects the entire family. As expressed by Mary Robinson in her poignant essay, "My Family Has Cancer" (see p. 56), each member will be dealing with stress and seeking ways to handle it.

- Don't expect to be able to handle the entire burden yourself. Seek, inform, and rely on allies or natural helpers—social workers, grandparents, close friends—to help you and your children through the ordeal.

- Inform other adults who are in frequent contact with your children of your situation, especially teachers, coaches, Scout leaders, and such. When your children are away from home, they still need to feel loved, protected, and cared for. Although your children may appear to be "toughing it out" when they are not with you, these key adults can do much to lessen the pain by listening, by encouraging, and simply by being a friend and protector.

- Find ways to lessen interruption of family time. Susan Stadnik provided daily "Andy Updates" to scores of family and friends using e-mail, thus reducing the number and impact of well-meaning but potentially intrusive phone calls (see p. 123).

- Try to preserve the children's basic routines (soccer games, school activities), which will help them maintain a level of emotional normalcy.

- Involve your children in illness-related activities, such as meetings with your doctor and shopping for wigs, if they show a readiness.

- Encourage family participation in preparation of special foods, if appropriate, such as macrobiotic meals.

- Find age-appropriate children's support groups. It is beneficial for children to learn that their situation is not unique. Other kids also have parents with cancer. Moreover, the professionals on staff and other children will help your children to "open up" and express their concerns.

Finally, monitor your own emotional, physical, spiritual, and optimistic levels. To be sure, it won't be easy. But it is helpful to remember that your children's level of tension will reflect yours. So, give thought to getting support for yourself.

Not every piece of advice will work in all situations. And it may be years before anyone knows how well your children have coped. As Dr. Wendy Harpham said in her thoughtful and comprehensive book, *When A Parent Has Cancer,* "Only time will tell the long-term effect of my illness on my children."

But you will find the right combination. And the result will be that your children will be better equipped to adapt to changing family dynamics and their changing senses of self, now and in the future.

Table Of Contents

Part 1

Professionals: Sharing Their Insight

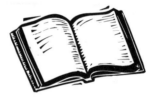

1

The Importance of Communicating with Your Kids About Cancer

by Madelyn Case, Ph.D. ⋆

The diagnosis of cancer in a parent has a severe impact on the entire family, shifting the focus and flow of time, money, energy, and emotional availability. Children and adolescents may see their importance diminished. They are faced with coping with a new entity, cancer, about which they know little. Communication between parent and child is important. The focus of this chapter is to offer guidance to parents: what, when and how to communicate, and why communication is important.

Child development experts agree that a child develops from egocentricity in infancy, to awareness of others in childhood, to sensitivity toward others in late teens and early adulthood. Many variations of development exist among families and cultures, but usually children are cared for, protected, controlled, and guided for many years, which emphasizes their value and importance.

Children grow up expecting safety and predictability in their lives. A diagnosis of cancer in either parent upsets those elements. The focus of the family shifts to the diagnosed par-

⋆ Dr. Case is herself a cancer survivor who, during her illness, was the mother of a teenage daughter.

ent. The world, as the child or adolescent has known it, has changed in a frightening way.

A parent wonders:

"What should I answer when my daughter asks, 'Are you going to die?'"

"I don't want to alarm my children, but I don't want to lie to them either. How much should I tell them?"

"I think my child understands, but I don't know. He never says anything to me about my cancer."

"I told my kids that I have cancer; now they just seem to act worse. What am I doing wrong?"

"What do I say to my kids?"

In almost all functional families, parents confronted with the diagnosis of cancer are concerned about their children. Facing their own mortality, often for the first time, the parents fear that one of them will die before the children are grown, that at least one of them will not be available to love, guide, and support the children through important milestones of their development. At the same time, despite these fears, parents want to reassure their children, to express hope, to be soothing and calm in the face of their children's anxiety. The questions above are the reflection of parental love and concern, sometimes to the point of desperation. "How do I instill in my child a sense of security, even in the face of danger?" we ask ourselves.

The Importance of Communication

Communication is inevitable whenever two or more persons are close. Although we tend to think of communication as speaking and listening, some of our most effective messages are nonverbal. Eye contact or lack of it, facial expressions, body posture, and gestures are common indicators of emotional and physical status, which we often interpret automatically without conscious thought. Even the suppression of verbal communication is a message—often perceived by another to mean, "What is not being spoken is in some way bad, fearful, or shameful."

Many ways exist to communicate with children. Every family has its unique set of dynamics, its own personality, so to speak. Children learn how to read and interpret messages of all kinds. When we send conflicting messages, confusion results. An example of conflicting messages might be a verbal message, "I'm going to be fine," accompanied by a nonverbal message of anxiety, pacing, and crying. Which will the child believe?

Information is very powerful because it helps a person feel more in control. Some denial is inevitable in coping with trauma, but we fight more effectively when we "know the enemy." Children are naturally curious and astonishingly resilient. Parents who are comfortable with their own emotions, open about imparting accurate factual information, and accepting of the natural responses and feelings of their children, will find that their children emulate them to the degree that they are able. That is, openness of the parent encourages openness in the children.

Except in cases of pervasive denial, lack of information often results in anxiety. When information is kept secret, the child still knows something is wrong. In the child's mind and imagination, there is a reason for secrecy. If the reason is not available, the child will invent one. Often the invented reason or story is much more anxiety-provoking than the real reason. For example, "It must be my fault, but they don't want me to know." The child feels compelled to hide this shameful "knowledge," thus lessening the chance of replacing it with reality, which would be less burdensome.

Sharing What Kind of Information and When?

The initial act of telling the child that a parent has been diagnosed with cancer is usually the task of one or both parents. The frightening nature of the word "cancer" can be diffused, emotionally, by an explanation of what cancer is, in simple terms; what treatment will be, if known; and the fact that most cancer is highly treatable. Along with these facts, it is very important to reassure children that they will continue to be loved and cared for on a continuing basis. Children also need to know that when they have questions or feel confused or unhappy, they can express their feelings to either parent.

Age is one indicator of development. Cognitive maturity indicates the capacity to hold and process information, to handle new vocabulary and concepts. At any age, children love new words and appreciate their parents including new terms (along with explanations) in discussions of cancer. Parents are often amused and gratified when they hear their children using the same new terms when explaining the situation to their friends.

Listening to Children's Questions and Comments

Stop! Take a breath! Listen! Parents often talk compulsively because of their own anxiety. Give children some time to ask questions. When you don't know the answer, say so. Reassure children that some questions don't really have answers, or that answers will be clearer as time passes, or that it would be a good question to ask the physician on a future visit.

Listen with the "third ear." Children's questions usually reflect feelings, and often those feelings are not easily expressed verbally. The child who asks if the parent who has cancer is going to die is probably saying a great deal more about fears of abandonment, loss of love, and his or her inability to cope with those feelings. Acknowledge those feelings for the child with reassurance of ongoing love. Point out that the very evident efforts of the medical people are based on their confidence and hope.

Keeping the Communication Door Open

When children or adolescents resist talking about cancer or listening to others' discussions, look at possible reasons.

Are your expectations too high? Children can handle only so much highly charged discussion; then they need a break.

Are your children afraid of expressing feelings? Look at your own openness in expressing feelings. They may be taking a cue from you. A feeling that is difficult to express is anger. Anger is a normal response to trauma, usually born out of unpredictability and a loss of control. Anger is often repressed by avoiding the anger-producing situation.

Avoiding discussion may be your child's way of maintaining at least partial denial. Sometimes parents unintentionally reinforce denial by making a rule of "Think only positive thoughts." Although hope and confidence are extremely important, a child may interpret such a rule as meaning not to discuss the disease at all.

Finding Allies and Resources

Many professionals are available: family, friends, groups, libraries, teachers, school counselors—even the Internet—to name a few. Other parents who have gone through the cancer experience, or who are doing so at the same time as you, are often helpful (as the essays in Part 2 illustrate). Both children and parents need to know: You don't have to do this alone!

Establishing Predictability

A certain progression of changes during cancer treatment is somewhat predictable. This information, presented early in the diagnosis and treatment-planning phase, helps children establish a sense of control over the emotional trauma that accompanies change, especially rapid and unexpected change. Chemotherapy, if part of the treatment plan, has predictable effects. Some of the most common are extreme fatigue, nausea, hair loss, irritability, and depression. When children are a part of the team to make the treatment results or disease symptoms as bearable as possible, they sense their own importance as helpers and healers. And who does not want to be perceived as a healer?

Assessing Yourself Emotionally

Probably the most important variable in communication with children is the emotional status of the parents. The stresses are great—physically, financially, and emotionally. Children often are called the barometers of the family: Their behavior reflects the emotional status of the family.

Parents may reduce their own emotional stress by using some of the resources mentioned above. In so doing, they may see reduced stress in their children.

Children manifest their emotions in many ways: whining, complaining, withdrawing, acting out, sleeping or eating differently, becoming physically ill. Often children do not really understand themselves or their behavior. To ask, "Why?" of children is often fruitless; they don't know. The circularity of the situation is apparent: Parents are upset, therefore children are upset; children respond in ways that neither parent nor child understands, leading to conflict, increased expectation for change, and increases emotional stress. If parents can find some relief for themselves, they are better able to understand and cope with their children's behavior.

Understanding the emotional roots of behavior does not always lead to a change in behavior, but chances for a healthier response increase if the child knows what is really bothering him or her. When parents remain attuned to their children's usual way of handling difficulties, they often can deduce what the underlying emotions may be. When children perceive that their parents are trying to understand—rather than reject—their behavior, they are reassured. Perhaps the most important thing a parent can communicate to a child is their awareness that something is bothering the child, that they want to understand and help, and that they love and care about the child.

In a support group for children whose parents have cancer, group leaders encourage the children to see themselves as heroes—figures who meet adversity, who get trampled, who are frustrated and depressed, who need to reach out to others in order to complete the journey. Really, every member of the cancer patient's family, parents and children alike, are heroes.

It has been my experience that many parents, confronted with the diagnosis of cancer and all that it implies, have been wonderfully wise in helping their children understand and cope with that anxiety-producing situation. Their methods and strategies have not all been the same, but they have been effective. Parents are vulnerable to seeing themselves as imperfect, and that vulnerability is increased by the advent of trauma in the family. Being true to ourselves and our values, and letting those aspects of ourselves be reflected in our behavior is, I think, the best we can do. Everyone is imperfect. Nothing works all the time, but hope, help, confidence, and desire will help solve many problems.

2

A Look Inside a Children's Support Group

*by Madelyn Case, Ph.D., Licensed Psychologist; Jeanne Currey, R.N., M.N.,
Clinical Nurse Specialist, Oncology Support Services, Porter Adventist Hospital,
Denver, CO, with Peter R. van Dernoot★*

Without a doubt, being a parent who has been diagnosed as having cancer is one of the cruelest situations one can encounter. Facing the possibility of dying without being able to raise one's children creates an enormous sense of failure.

In 1993, as we at Porter Adventist Hospital in Denver, Colorado, treated our adult cancer patient-parents, mostly women with breast cancer, we began to sense a real concern of theirs: the effect of cancer on their children and the availability of support resources. We became aware that we ought to be doing something to stabilize the emotions of the parents' children. Our patients would ask, "Do our children really understand the seriousness of the situation? One minute they're sad, the next minute they go out and play!"

Children know something isn't right. But depending on their age, they may not have the vocabulary or the insight to express their fears. Moreover, their needs may be missed by overwhelmed parents and by medical staff concerned with treating the cancer patient. Still, most children will grieve

* This article was the basis of a story that appeared in Oncology Times, April 1999. The authors hope this account will motivate parents to consider finding a support program for their children and inspire professionals to start similar programs in their facilities.

appropriately if adults don't confuse them. Although an ill person becomes, of necessity, more self-centered, children can be helped to see beyond this crisis and beyond themselves.

Children have many reactions to a parent's illness. As adolescents, this may take the form of rebelling, showing temper, and getting "mouthy." Additionally, as they try to make sense of or cope with their parent's cancer, children of all ages may display some of the following:

- Refusal to talk about cancer

- Over-responsible behavior

- Sleep disturbances

- Significant changes in school or social behaviors

- Withdrawal

- Verbalized fears

- Clinging

- Physical complaints

As we explored the possibilities of developing a children's support group, we knew the questions, but not the answers: "What should be done? What ages of children are we thinking about? Where will we get the funding and the time?"

Setting Goals

In thinking through the dynamics experienced by our patient families, we determined that our primary focus was to be the children. We would help them to recognize and to understand their feelings and to become aware of how they were expressing them externally. We hoped they would then be able to bridge their inner feelings with their outward behavior in a healthy manner. A secondary objective was to help the parents understand and interpret their children's behavior. Although many parents may try to treat family activities as "normal," they need to be aware that their child is still thinking about the hard issues, such as, "What if Mom dies?"

Thus, the goals of the children's support group were set:

- Provide a safe, helpful environment where children are encouraged to express their feelings.

- Create a place for a child to be a child—to experience fun, support, and continuity of life—apart from the illness.

- Improve relations between cancer patients and their children, thereby reducing any guilt and anxiety in the children.

- Help parents understand their children's adaptive behavior as a reaction to illness.

Just as we were conceptualizing the project, we were dramatically reminded of its need. A member of our staff was diagnosed with breast cancer. During the next several months, as a single parent with an adopted daughter then 16, she went through the emotional and physical agony that has entered the lives of millions of women worldwide: chemotherapy treatments, a mastectomy, hair loss, sickness, and ultimately, recovery. As the months went by and her activity moved into "routine" check-ups, she noticed significant behavioral changes in her daughter. What had previously been a "sweet and caring child" became one who threw temper tantrums, slamming doors and mouthing off.

After one particular follow-up visit to the doctor and her daughter's temperamental outburst, she asked, "What in the world is wrong with you?" expecting the answer would be related to a teenage boyfriend problem. "Mom," she said, "you don't understand that every time you come home from a follow-up cancer check-up, I never know what you're going to have to tell me." Clearly, our patients and their children needed help.

Finding Resources

With our goals established, the intensity of our project increased as we explored funding possibilities. Fortunately, the project was recognized as deserving financial support by substantial outside organizations. Funding for the first year was provided by the Susan G. Komen Foundation. Year two was funded by Boston Market. Ongoing financial support has been provided by the Porter Foundation and the Porter Adventist Hospital Auxiliary.

Additionally, the in-kind support from Porter Adventist Hospital—office space, secretarial services, mailing and postage expenses—and a growing core of volunteer staff have helped to keep the annual expenses relatively low, in the $12,000 to $15,000 range.

Program Content

With initial funding secured, the Support Group for Children of Parents with Cancer was launched. The program, entirely free and available to any family in the area, has since served dozens of kids ages 6 to 16, helping them to cope with the trauma of a parent's cancer. (The program is now called Kids Alive!—Support for Children of Parents with Cancer.)

Each program spans nine months. In the process, children and adolescents—whether exhibiting maladaptive behaviors or not—benefit from two-and a-half hour group sessions where they experience support and help through a wide variety of fun and interesting activities, including winter sports outings, hiking, drama, art, movement, relaxation, imagery, and discussion.

Our calendar of activities is as follows:

October

This is the first session and activities are chosen to help establish friendship and trust. Later in the session an oncologist explains, in children's terms, the nature of cancer. Recently, he showed a series of slides on how he cured a tiger's cancer at the Denver Zoo. Talk about interest!

November

"A Hero's Journey." This session is designed to set the tone, to provide the underpinning for the overall program. Children hear a story dealing with loss. They then act out a situation where they find themselves in the belly of a whale, and they have to figure out how to escape. This requires their developing new friends and support—"allies"—and working together.

Then they find themselves on a "Road of Trials," where they must slay a dragon, earn a wish, and get knighted.

In the process, they learn there are many ways to become a "hero" and, equally important, most heroes don't achieve success by themselves; they must trust others and rely on support from allies. In the time and space of the "hero's event," they become highly energized and motivated to help each other, learning new interpersonal skills in the process. Although most kids do not come in with a "woe is me" attitude, through group discussions they begin to express deep feelings. Ongoing discussions follow on how their ill parents behave, how it affects them, and where they can go for help, in other words, allies.

Because this is just the second group session, many children are hesitant and afraid when they enter. By the time they leave, however, they have formed new friendships in a unique peer group, and they begin to talk openly about their feelings.

December

An art therapist leads a session where the children create art that reflects how they feel. In one situation, the therapist, a cancer survivor herself, shows the children a collage she had made depicting how she had once felt, using abstract items such as nails, wire, and pieces of metal.

Skillfully, she suggests to the children that feelings are not always easily expressed, and they are not always "warm and fuzzy." The children easily interpret the art, observing that life can have sharp, rough edges to it. This leads to helpful discussion.

January

Children hear and discuss the short book, *The Fall of Freddie the Leaf*, by the late Leo Buscaglia, Ph.D. This helps them think through changing seasons and personal loss.

Older children then do "family sculpting," creating interactive family portraits depicting the family's cancer situation. Younger children participate in a puppet activity reflecting their family experience. Discussions evolve: "How did you hear about your mom's/dad's cancer?" "What were you thinking when you heard about it?" "How do you feel now?"

February

A music therapist takes the children through an interactive group activity using various percussion items as rain stick, drums, bells, and tone blocks. After groups of children master some basic skills, she then melds them into a mini-orchestra. Voila! They've learned what can be achieved through the combination of individual skills and team effort. This then leads into a catch-up discussion on their feelings.

March

A mountain outing takes place. The children spend a weekend at Snow Mountain Ranch, a YMCA mountain camp in Colorado, where they experience wall-climbing with belaying and rappelling (while learning a lot about trusting and support!), snowball fights, roller skating, sledding, swimming, a campfire with ghost stories and s'mores, and other activities.

A number of parents go to help provide support. For other parents, it provides a much-needed break. Their children are able to call home if they feel the need.

April

An art therapist encourages the kids to paint on muslin, a quilt square reflecting something that has been important to them in the group, which gets sewn into a master quilt.

May

The children view the completed quilt, reflecting their combined efforts and impressions.

Then, depending on the weather, they draw posters with the theme of preventing and curing cancer, or they bike and rollerblade in a nearby park.

Finally, the children plan their last session, which will

include their parents. By now, the children have become much more confident in themselves and in the group, talking openly about what has been important and memorable to them during the year. Somewhat surprisingly, in some cases their thoughts have gone from normal self-centered attitudes to ones expressing concern for others, such as, "Can we do something to help other needy people?"

June

The final session: A Kids and Parents event. Children talk with their parents about what they've learned and how they feel. Then, it's picnic time for all!

The Outcomes

Without exception, children who exhibited behavioral patterns of concern (and many who hadn't) have brightened into happier, enthusiastic kids. They clearly have loosened up, discussing more easily and openly how they feel with their newfound friends and their parents. Moreover, a new sense of confidence and selflessness is evident in the children at the June session: Most of them want to come back the following year to be helpers—to be a buddy to someone else! One young boy expressed his enthusiasm, saying, "Next year, I'll bring my little sister. She's too young now, but she should come next year." And she did!

The parents report that their children are much more able to talk about cancer and its impact on the family. They say that the children's having a place to look forward to where they can talk with peers who are handling the same hurt enables them to loosen up. One mother, whose family had moved out-of-state after the children's father died of cancer early in the program, sensed this and drove her children a total of 1,200 miles back to Colorado to make sure they could participate in the Snow Mountain Ranch outing. One mother knew that the program had worked and that her son had reached a "major milestone" when he encouraged: "Mom, it's okay if you don't wear your wig."

What the Kids Say

HOW DOES THE PARENT WITH CANCER ACT?

They sleep all day

Quiet

Their medication is next to them

Grumpy

Never comes downstairs

Never walks

Sits around and watches TV

Asks to be left alone

Sighs a lot and rubs temples

Gets calls from the hospital

Receives medical aides at the house

Tired

Sometimes I have to stay with other people

They are gone a lot

They complain

They ask you to do a lot of stuff

They ask you to be quiet

They eat special foods or they don't eat much

Ask you to go play outside or in your bedroom

They sleep in a special kind of bed

They get a special room in the house

HOW DO YOU FEEL?

Depressed	Worried
Sad	Scared
Guilty	Sheltered
Mixed up	Lonely
Helpless	Nervous
Angry	Confused
Stressed	Numb

You don't want to play with anyone

You feel like you want to help a lot

You don't want to leave Mom or Dad because they might need you

You wish it had never happened

You need support

You don't want to be separated

Afraid that Mom or Dad won't live

You don't feel safe

Afraid of going to an orphanage

You picture things happening that you don't like

It feels like you need to be comforted

You feel like you want to beat someone up

You feel like you have to grow up really fast

Sometimes you feel like you've lost faith in God

You sometimes get grossed out

You feel like you want to be in bed all the time

You feel calm—not hyped up

You feel like you don't know what's happening

It feels like it's your fault

You feel like you want to get on your skateboard and get away

HOW HAS LIFE CHANGED?

You have to take more responsibility

You gain a better respect for life

There isn't any time to do what you want to do

The family is eating more healthily

People are always taking you everywhere

You do more family stuff

You feel sad more often

You don't get to do as much because of the family's money situation

You have to do more stuff by yourself

You learn a lot more about disease

You learn to live with going to other people's houses

People come to your house to take care of you

You sometimes forget about your parent's cancer

You talk about cancer but still don't understand it

You get to talk to your parents more often

You stay home with your parents most of the time

You think about your mom and dad more often

You miss your parents more when you're not with them

You get to do more stuff with your parents

WHO OR WHAT ARE YOUR ALLIES?

The doctor

Your grandparents

Other relatives

Siblings

Your mom's friend

Your teacher

The school's student counselor

Your pets

Your notebook

A reading book

Spiritual

Stuffed animals

HOW DO YOU HELP YOURSELF?

Help out around the house

Ask a lot of questions

Talk about it with Mom, Dad, and the doctor

Know when Mom or Dad has treatment

Get answers

3

Sharing the Journey with Your Child

by Peggy Anne Murphy, L.M.S.W., Cancer Care, Inc.; Les Gallo-Silver, L.C.S.W.R., Cancer Care, Inc.; Stacy Kramer, L.M.S.W., Cancer Care, Inc.

The most difficult thing for any parent to do is to tell their child that they have cancer. All parents want to protect their children. It is natural to want to protect your child from your cancer. The best way to protect your child is also the hardest, which is to include them. Children need and depend on their parents so very much that they easily pick up that something is wrong. Left to their own devices, children often believe that something terrible has happened and that it is their fault.

How and when you will tell your child will be different for each parent. Only you know your child and the relationship you share well enough to decide the how and the when. The experiences shared in the group help you think through these decisions with more information and clarity. Your children will have the comfort and reassurances they need at their fingertips if it is possible for you and/or your spouse to be the people who share the news with them. If you feel tearful when you do talk with your children, consider letting them comfort you. Telling your children about your cancer is an opportunity to help them develop empathy and compassion. It is an opportunity for them to demonstrate how much they love you. You will read how all the children in this book wanted to help and contribute in some way in their parent's fight against cancer. Sharing your journey as you meet the challenge of your cancer will connect you in a deeper emotional way to your children. This new deeper emotional connection will comfort you as much as it comforts them.

As a parent, your cancer and its treatment are a complex journey. How to share that journey with your children raises many questions and concerns.

Can I still perform my normal activities such as working, taking care of the house and my children? Should my children know about the cancer diagnosis? What should they know? Will information scare my children? What do I do if I can't answer a question? How can I still protect them? What if I cry? Why does my child seem so angry? Why is my child more withdrawn? How come sleep time has become such a problem? Parents seek the answers to these questions because they love their children so very much.

In order to answer parents' questions and respond to their concerns, the Children's Services Committee at CancerCare developed a two-hour program which is titled: We're Talking About It™. The goal of the program is to help parents problem-solve about how best to help their children. The program helps parents find creative, soothing, and comforting ways of helping their child with their feelings about their parent's cancer and the changes in the family caused by cancer. This helps parents by enhancing their role as the person who takes care of their child's needs even in times of stress.

We're Talking About It™ consists of group activities for the children, while their parents are in their own separate "talking" group next door. The parents share their feelings about parenting while in treatment, their worries about their children's reactions to the change in their energy level and availability and the change in the family's routines. Parents come away with confidence that no matter how powerfully felt a cancer diagnosis may be, it does not have the power to take away their ability to be a great parent. Parents are the experts on their children. The mantra for the program and for all work with children and families comes from Mr. Rogers: "Whatever is human is mentionable and whatever is mentionable is manageable."

The activities for children, ages 6 to 12, are divided into simple healing exercises that help the children feel connected to each other and supported by one another. The activities focus on reaching five specific healing goals:

1) To help the children begin to connect to each other. To help the children feel safe and secure with the group leaders.

2) To provide accurate, age-appropriate information about cancer.

3) To identify and normalize common feelings and to identify appropriate ways to express feelings.

4) To help children find and name the people in their life who can comfort and help them. To encourage children to reach out to the people who will help them.

5) To encourage families to see themselves as part of a larger community, including the group they formed through this program. To demonstrate to both children and adults that they are connected to others and that they can take that connection with them.

The Game Show of Knowledge

This is an example of one of the activities. This activity will be easy for you to use at home with your family.

Goals: To provide accurate, age-appropriate information about cancer and to correct misinformation about cancer.

The family can be put into two teams as designated by a red or blue dot on their name tag. The parents can choose categories and then read the questions to the teams. Each team then huddles together to discuss a question and answer, in case the first team that goes gets the question wrong. A parent will help with the discussion, ensuring that all who want to say something in the small group have a chance. Points are given. Teams take turns choosing and answering until time is up. Everyone is a winner and each child is given a small prize.

The names of the categories and some sample true/false questions and answers:

Q: It's never a child's fault, when a parent gets cancer.

A: TRUE

Q: Cancer can be caught like a cold.

A: FALSE

Q: You can't make cancer go away by being good or bad.

A: TRUE

Q: It is okay to feel different from other kids at school when your parent has cancer.

A: TRUE

Q: Sometimes children get angry because their parent has cancer.

A: TRUE

Q: Cancer is not contagious. You can't get cancer by hugging, kissing, touching, or using the same dishes or spoons/forks.

A: TRUE

Q: Talking to others about your feelings is a way to feel better.

A: TRUE

Q: You talk to _____ (parents, teachers, grandparents, counselors, aunts, uncles) when you have big feelings.

A: TRUE

HAVING FUN

Q: We still celebrate holidays and birthdays when parents are sick with cancer.

A: TRUE

Q: It is ok to laugh when a parent has cancer.

A: TRUE

TREATMENTS

Q: Chemotherapy makes many people need to sleep more.

A: TRUE

Q: Chemotherapy can make your hair fall out.

A: TRUE

Q: Chemotherapy causes many side effects; one of them is that the parent may be cranky.

A: TRUE

CANCER HELPERS

Q: The nurse takes the parent's temperature and gives them medicine.

A: TRUE

Q: Parents with cancer may not be able to do all the things they used to because they are feeling tired. _____(Grandparents, Aunts/Uncles or Home Attendants) can come to the house to help with the parent wash up, get dressed, and eat.

A: TRUE

The Parents' Talking Group

The parents' talking group meets while the children are engaged in the first four activities and they join the children for the fifth activity. The group is an education and problem-solving opportunity. The information listed below is some of the wisdom shared in the groups.

For parents of school-age children:

1. Children need accurate, age-appropriate information about cancer.

2. Given their age and prior experience with serious illness in the family, parents need to spend their energy communicating with their children. Some children need several short talks so that they can adjust to the information gradually.

3. Children must know that no matter how they have been behaving or what they have been thinking, they did not do anything to cause the cancer.

4. Children need to be reminded about the other people in their lives who care about them, their support system, including the other parent, relatives, clergy, coaches, friends, and the parent's healthcare team.

5. Children must be allowed to participate and make a contribution to the parent's care by giving them age appropriate tasks, i.e., bringing a glass of water or reading to the parent.

6. Children need to be encouraged to have and to express feelings, even the ones that are uncomfortable. They also need to know that it is ok to say, "I don't want to talk right now."

7. Children need to be assured that their needs are still important and that they will be cared for, even if you can't always provide them with the care directly.

8. Children need to have an explanation of the treatment plan and what this will mean for them.

9. Parents need to show their children lots of love and affection. They need to know that although things are different, your love for them has not changed.

For parents of teenage children:

1. Teenagers are unpredictable. When a teenager learns that their parent has cancer, there is no correct response. Recognize and respect that there are a variety of responses your teenager may have. Keep in mind that your teenager may be uncomfortable with some or all of their feelings and thoughts about your cancer.

2. Teenagers want detailed information. This is especially true when it comes to information about diagnosis, treatment and prognosis, including the correct terminology. They may seek out further information on their own in addition to what you have provided.

3. Teenagers need to know the truth and may feel particularly sensitive to information that they feel is incomplete or inaccurate.

4. Teenagers need privacy. This need for privacy does not mean that your teen feels alone. They may or may not want to talk about the experience with their family. Reassure your teenager that they can receive support from other sources, i.e., an aunt, grandparent, a friend's parent, a teacher, clergy person, or another member of the extended family.

5. Teenagers often discuss, write, and reflect, going where their thoughts lead them. Encourage your teenagers to share these feelings and concerns. They can also channel this energy to athletics, journaling, or other creative arts.

6. Teenagers who want to contribute to care-giving should be allowed to participate in tasks that respect that they are not adults and yet no longer young children.

7. Encourage teenagers who want to accompany their family member to treatment in order to see the facility and meet the treatment team. This can be helpful in terms of feeling more control about how your medical care is provided.

8. Teenagers need consistency. Make an effort to ensure that they will still attend normal activities and social events.

9. Teenagers struggle with the need for independence. A parent's illness may make this more difficult. Encourage your teenager to spend time with friends in age-appropriate activities as well as with family.

10. Teenagers are often self-conscious. Much of the typical teenager 'angst' comes from feeling unique and misunderstood. A teenager whose parent has cancer may feel even more different. Help your teenager to understand that there are others going through a similar experience; you might suggest that they participate in a support group, peer-to-peer network, or online chat room.

Each child will cope in their own way. Some will want to write down their thoughts, others may want to draw, while others will develop little skits with dolls or action figures. The interest you show in their way of coping will help them feel protected and loved. Cherish each crayoned picture, each poem, story, or skit. These are all meant to help you as much as it helps your child.

Involving your children's teachers and other adults in your child's life will help create a community of caring for them. Teachers, guidance counselors, school psychologists, and social workers can become key members of your team that helps your child where they spend so much of their time. Consider involving the parents of your child's friends and playmates. The comfort you display by reaching out to them will serve as a model of how you want them to interact with you and with your child.

Parenting is more of an art than a science. Your children are your life's masterpieces. Everything you give them with love and sincerity helps them to become kind and giving people. Cancer is frightening and devastating; yet helping your children cope with your cancer can be a way for you to show how much you care about and love them. It will be the hardest thing you have ever done, and this book and the personal stories and programs contained in it will help you do it the best way for you and your child.

4

Kids Count's "Chemo Bear" Hits the Road to Meet Special Needs

by Sam Harris, M. Div., Patient Advocate, Erlanger Cancer Center,

Chattanooga, Tennessee

It's 5:45 a.m. in early spring, and "Chemo Bear" and I are sitting in the parking lot of Channel 12, our local CBS affiliate, awaiting Janet Kramer-Mai, the Breast Center Educator for the Erlanger Cancer Center in Chattanooga, Tennessee. What brings us out on a cool morning just to do a four-minute spot on "News 12 This Morning"?

When Janet was hired to develop the role of the Oncology Educator for the Erlanger Cancer Center, she had difficulty finding appropriate resources for patients and their families. Not only was there nothing here in Chattanooga, but she could not find any resources in nearby hospitals in Atlanta, Knoxville, Nashville or Memphis. Surprised by the lack of support, Janet would ask why, and often heard the recurring phrase: "Kids are resilient; they will bounce back just fine!" This was really disturbing to her; kids *are* resilient, but she felt that they needed the proper tools to help them cope.

After a great deal of research, Janet found a helpful group in California and began the journey to launch a program at Erlanger in mid-October 2001. This would be an event in the cancer center featuring tours of each of the treatment areas and a time allocated for the kids and parents to ask questions and familiarize themselves with the "treatment world."

However, ten days before the kick-off, Janet was diagnosed with breast cancer. Fortunately, co-workers and her sister all pitched in to see that the event went off without a hitch and 13 children attended that first gathering. Janet, with three young boys, realized even more how important it was to provide coping skills for children dealing with a loved one diagnosed with cancer. Cancer not only affects the person diagnosed, but has a major impact on the entire family.

She had done some marketing for the group in area schools and met the guidance counselor at one of our private elementary schools. The counselor was working with an 8-year-old whose mother had a brain tumor. The counselor started bringing the child to the group meetings at the Erlanger Cancer Center, and my predecessor went to the school to meet with the child after their mother died. Unfortunately, after a couple of years, the program ceased to function effectively, with only a few students attending, and sometimes—none.

In September of 2004, I was hired as the Patient Advocate for Oncology in Erlanger's Cancer Center. My primary responsibility was to provide emotional and spiritual (working with our Pastoral Care Office) encouragement for cancer patients and their families. I inherited three support programs, one of which was "Kids Count." During those early fall months, we tried to revive the program with little success.

In October 2004, Janet received material about a scheduled workshop sponsored by The Children's Treehouse Foundation in Denver, Colo. I also was given a copy of Peter van Dernoot's book, **_Helping Your Children Cope with Your Cancer, A Guide For Parents And Families._** After reading Peter's book, I was convinced that there was much for us to learn in order to rebuild this important outreach to children. The work shop was titled "CLIMB: Children's Lives Include Moments of Bravery." Janet and our Oncology Administrator, Linda Smith, suggested that I attend this training in December, which had 18 participants from major hospitals throughout the country.

Upon returning from Denver, I wrote a proposal to adopt the CLIMB model and presented it to our Leadership Team. We were given approval to proceed with the new program. New brochures were printed, and all of our craft supplies were donated by children in one of our churches. Our newly revamped program was also publicized on radio and television spots.

Now back to 5:45 a.m. on that cool spring morning. Janet and I, along with "Chemo Bear," had been invited to discuss our new Kids Count program in a four-minute segment. A few weeks later, we were given another opportunity to publicize the program during a five-minute slot on the local ABC affiliate. Our telephone number scrolled across the screen, and upon returning to the hospital, we waited for the calls to come in. We had received great, free publicity reaching thousands of people, but no one called!

Our initial startup was disappointing, but not discouraging; we had traditionally held Kids Count at Erlanger, and sometimes, at the Ronald McDonald House across the street. Several factors faced us when we attempted to host these programs on our campus: (1) what do parents do while their children are participating in the program? (2) How do we compete with soccer, baseball, football, etc, and (3) How do we address the fact that many parents are simply too tired to drive their children to these support programs? During our initial signup period, no one registered.

The school guidance counselor, with whom Janet had previously worked, had been counseling a number of children whose parents had cancer, and she contacted our Resource Center for help. It was then we decided that if the children couldn't come here, we could take Kids Count to them, and that's what we did. This concept was approved by the principal, and we started our school visit program with five children. In May of 2005, we finished our first six weeks' program with them and took them on two summer outings. It worked so well, that the school officials invited us back in the fall and have recommended Kids Count to other private elementary schools in Chattanooga. This year, 2006, we are currently working with seven students at the elementary school, have launched a second program, at a small boutique in north Georgia, to meet the needs of our Georgia patients. We will begin a third program at another private elementary school, followed by a fourth at one of our local malls. Our Leadership Team comprises Janet, Carla Goette, a bereavement coordinator with a local hospice program, and me. "Chemo Bear" is a large teddy bear who often accompanies us to our meetings. When the children visit Erlanger's Radiation and Infusion areas of the hospital, he "receives" chemo and radiation helping to dispel fears they might have about their parents' treatment.

How beneficial has this in-school program been to the schools thus far? I quote from the guidance counselor:

"I want to thank you, Sam, Janet and Carla for bringing your wonderful program into our school setting. In the past, I have worried about how to service the children with sick parents. You all have been a prayer answered! During the past 1-2 years, the need for group counseling for these children in our school has been great. One of the concerns in the past has been how the caregiver would get the children to the meetings. In fact, about two years ago I personally drove one of our students to the Ronald McDonald house and took her home afterward, – so she could attend the meetings. So, now with six children affected, know that I am very thankful that you have brought the program to us. When I asked the kids what the group has meant to them, some of the responses included: 'It helps us learn about cancer' (from Madison) and 'It helps us to know that we aren't the only ones at school with a sick parent' (from Keegan). I personally believe the group does this, and more. It gives them a support system, an arena to discuss, understand, and explore feelings and experiences. They can interact by crafts, stories, and other "fun" activities. The groups are structured so that they aren't always sad, depressing meetings – they really do enjoy getting together to talk and do an activity. But at the same time, they have been so good at recognizing their feelings of confusion, sadness, worry, anger. So, on behalf of our entire elementary school (teachers, students, and families), I thank you for your service, for your caring personality and for your program. I look forward to our groups this year!"

—Jennifer Greer, Boyd-Buchanan School Elementary Counselor

Soon, several of our children at Boyd-Buchanan will be "graduating" from the program since their mothers have gone into remission. We are planning a special party and cake for them, but they will not leave the program; our plans are to use them as helpers with some of the younger children.

Our goal is to reach as many of the schools in our area as possible over the next several years. At this point, the private schools, we have 16, are more open to this program than the public schools. In time, we believe the public schools will recognize the need for their children due to the success we are having in the private institutions. We are happy to share both our successes and failures and welcome any inquiries regarding our programs using the CLIMB model. For us, going to the schools and areas where children live has proven to be a unique opportunity to help them learn coping skills when cancer impacts their families.

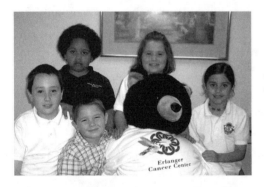

Chemo Bear with some of the children in the Kids Count program.

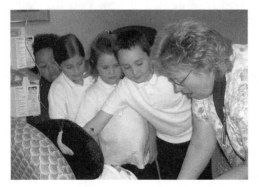

Brave Chemo Bear receives an injection as the concerned kids look on. It doesn't hurt a bit!

Part II

Parents: Helping Their Kids Cope

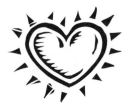

5
Unconditional Love

by Peggy Peters

I am the mother of two children, Maggie, 6, and Amy Grace, 3; and I am a breast cancer survivor. In the winter months, I am a supervisor in the Vail/Beaver Creek Ski School in Colorado. In the summer months, I enjoy being a full-time mother.

I discovered a lump in my breast while nursing my youngest daughter, who was 8 months old at the time. I remember the first thing I said after my doctor told me the news: "I can't have cancer. I have two children to raise."

From the very beginning, my thoughts went to how I was going to get through this and still raise my children the way I dreamed of raising them. My greatest fear was that I would not survive. I had known only one person who had had breast cancer, and she died, leaving three small children and her husband.

This was a difficult time. My husband had just bought a new business that brought with it many pleasures and demands. It was also 10 days before Christmas, approaching my busy time on the mountain. And, of course, we were anticipating Santa's arrival very soon!

I went on to have a mastectomy and chemotherapy; four courses of one chemical agent followed by another.

After my surgery, I showed Maggie, then 3, my scar. She was very interested in what was happening, although she couldn't really understand what was going on. She called it my "scrape" (and still does) and asked me every day if my scrape was getting better.

I was worried that she would be scared and bewildered when I lost my hair. These were the feelings I was anticipating myself. I decided to make the hair loss something we would all prepare for in a fun way.

I wanted Maggie to be a part of my hair loss "adventure," so I planned a hair-cutting party for us all and a few close friends. We all gathered at my home after I had recovered from my first round of chemo. Everyone had a great time chopping away at my shoulder-length hair. Maggie especially enjoyed cutting it and felt very important with grown-ups that night. I asked my regular hairdresser to be there that night so she could shape things up so I could enjoy my first experience with short hair— even if it would last for only another 10 days.

When my hair did fall out, it didn't seem to affect my daughter at all. She had a great time trying on my wig and helping me with my scarves. She was always so loving on those days when I would break down, and she would shower me with her hugs and kisses.

Since my children were so small when I was going through my treatment, they weren't aware that I could die from cancer. What made the biggest impression on me, though, was their reaction to me as I went through my changes in appearance.

Amy Grace would react to me with the same smiles, the same needs, and the same love whether I had my wig on, my scarves or hats, or had my bare head showing.

The thing that touched my heart the most was the fact that "who I was" to them was not my hair, or eyebrows, or chest. We connected in our love with our eyes and touch and words. They already knew the things that mattered most.

My children gave me the most important gift I have ever received: the gift of unconditional love.

In so many ways, cancer gave me many gifts. And for that I am truly thankful.

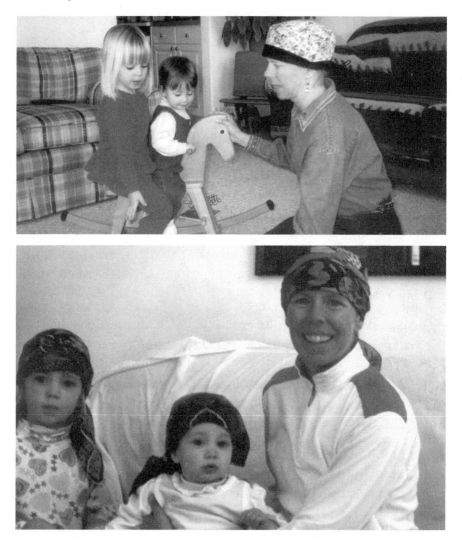

Peggy, with Maggie, left, two years old, and Amy, ten months old.

6

A Little Understanding Goes a Long Way

by Maia Rogers, M.P.P., M.P.H.

I keep a small, dirty, crumpled piece of paper in my journal and look at it often. It's from two years ago, when I was battling breast cancer and my son Eddy was three and in preschool. His teachers had helped him write a "fill in the blank" letter to me entitled, "All About Mommy." He wrote about my favorite color, my favorite food (goldfish—which is actually his favorite food), and what I liked to play with (according to him, cars). The part that really opened my heart said this, "My mommy likes to sleep cause she's really sick, but she's feeling better."

I started to cry. Despite our efforts to maintain a normal life while I battled breast cancer, it became clear to me that Eddy, and surely our then five-year-old daughter Caitlin, were affected by the cancer. Although the cancer was happening to me, I knew that this crisis for me was also a life-changing event for my young children.

As I look back on that time, it doesn't surprise me that the kids knew that something was going on. When I was first diagnosed with invasive ductal carcinoma, my husband and I moved right into research mode because of our science backgrounds. We spent hours on the internet, on the phone with experts, and poring over pages of materials. I was on the phone a lot. I cried a lot. The kids saw this and were worried.

They heard "cancer" and "surgery" and "hospital" and "doctor" and lots of other medical terms that surely sounded ominous to their little ears. Sometimes, they heard Mommy crying that she didn't want to die. I can't imagine how scary that must have sounded to them.

During the next six months, as I underwent two major surgeries and chemotherapy, the kids' normal routine was disrupted. My parents came from Hawaii to help us care for them. We scheduled play dates so that they would get outside and have some fun and I could get some quiet. Friends brought dinners. The kids were told to be quiet so that I could rest. I had been their primary caregiver and now I was in bed, too sore to give them decent hugs, too sick to read them stories, unable to play with them as they were accustomed.

My husband, Jed, and I tried the best we could to talk to the children about what was going on. We decided that they should hear the truth and the correct terminology from us rather than rumors and half truths from their friends or ours. "Mommy is sick," we said. "She has cancer. Cancer is bad cells in your body. The doctors are helping her to get the bad cells out of her body." We told them about chemotherapy. "Chemotherapy is medicine that will fight the bad cells. But it will make her tired and her hair will fall out." We found a few books that talked about cancer, but we knew that the kids continued to have questions and we didn't have all the answers.

Jed and I were worried. How was this experience going to affect our children? It was clear that they were confused and stressed. Caitlin started having major tantrums. She regressed to having accidents in school. Eddy was hitting kids at his preschool. We asked ourselves, "Is this normal?" and "What can we do to help them?" We needed help.

We started to look for resources to help our children deal with cancer. We found several support groups that were aimed at older children ages 7 and up. However, we could not find anything for young children. We were told that the kids were too young to process what was going on. But we could see them processing every day. Finally, we saw a notice for the KIND program on the bulletin board at the Rocky Mountain Cancer Center. The notice described a group program to support children under age 7 who had a parent going through cancer. We immediately signed up.

Our hope for the support group was that we would get the information we needed to help our children through my cancer without irreparable harm. We hoped that the kids would talk about how they felt, their fears, their hopes. We wanted help talking to the kids about cancer. We wanted to give them just the right amount of information, not too much and not too little. Perhaps most importantly, we wanted to know that they would be okay.

The KIND program, now called CLIMB (Children's Lives Include Moments of Bravery), at the University of Colorado Cancer Center, is a six-week program that involved therapists who did hands-on projects involving dance, puppetry, drawing, horticulture, music, and play. Parents and children were separated for half an hour and then brought together to end the session.

The kids started to talk about cancer. They talked about Mommy dying. They fought the cancer with play swords and tenderly played house. They dramatized our experience with cancer; putting on plays about a flower being planted and reborn. They drew butterflies. Remarkably, despite the heavy weight of the topic the kids were discussing, they always ended the session happy. At the end of each evening, they could describe how they were feeling by picking from a stack of yellow faces showing different emotions. They always chose, "I feel happy" or "I feel silly."

My children may not remember the KIND program. They may not even remember these past two years that we battled cancer. But I know that the KIND program helped me help them get through a very difficult and painful time. Without these unique resources, we would not have been able to understand their needs at this complex time in our lives. Sometimes a little understanding goes a long way toward healing. I encourage you to find a professional, support group for your children as you go through your cancer journey.

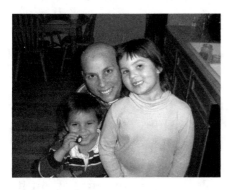

Maia Rogers during chemo treatment, with her children, Eddy, age 3, and Caitlin, age 5.

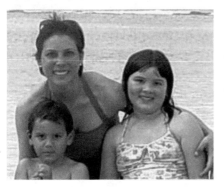

Ten months after the end of treatment, Maia and the children in Hawaii.

7

"Mom, I Lost It Today!"

by Karen Sturm, M.S., M.F.T./A.T. Intern

My daughter and I were diagnosed with cancer.

Don't think for a minute that it was happening to just me. We were both affected. I was experiencing the physical part; she was experiencing the emotional part, just as strongly as when I was crying over mouth sores. She emotionally felt the stick of the needles, the nausea, and most importantly, the fear.

Claire is a brave soul, and in some cases braver than me. When I was sick from treatment, exhausted from attending my last graduate classes, writing my thesis, working internship hours at an elementary school (while bald, I must say), and flying from California to Illinois for my chemotherapy every 3 weeks, Claire endured it all. The pressure mounted onto her shoulders and I was helpless to do anything about it. Was I helpless because of the illness? You better believe it. I made choices to stay busy to keep myself sane. Yet, what I forgot during this time, and with the experience of being a marriage and family therapy intern and art therapist, CLAIRE WAS SUFFERING. She never said it. She never complained. But one day while she was at school, she called me in tears, "Mom, I lost it today! I ran out of school because my mind went blank on a test. I knew the answers, but my mind was blank!" The weight of her unexpressed experiences, thoughts, fears, and anxiety came to fruition, and she cried with friends around while she sat on a curb next to her high school.

It wasn't until the month AFTER my treatment was over that I began discussing in length what my cancer was all about. When I heard her words being uttered, "Wow, I didn't know THAT!" did it really begin to sink in. What I hadn't done was to include Claire into my experience, and the result of that was increased anxiety and torment for her.

I break down in tears at this moment thinking about it. While doing a literature review for my qualifying thesis, I learned what children go through during a parent's bout with cancer, whether in a large family or small one like mine. In the process, I learned about The Children's Treehouse Foundation. And after having long conversations with Peter van Dernoot, Founder and Executive Director, regarding their support groups for children, CLIMB (Children's Lives Included Moments of Bravery), I am dedicating my career to helping children, adolescents and families in similar situations.

Yeah, and I also dedicate my efforts on behalf of my incredible daughter, Claire Andrea Sturm, who deserves the world.

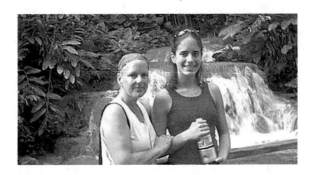

Karen Sturm, during treatment, with her daughter, Claire.

8

Do It With Love, and All Else Is Irrelevant

by Becky Richards, R. N.

I certainly hope that what I have to share is helpful, but at the same time, I feel each person is her own best help when she is stricken with cancer. You alone know what is right, best, and prudent for your child. The answer must come from you. That is what your child wants. That is what your child needs.

On my twelfth birthday, my mother was diagnosed with inflammatory carcinoma of the breast. She was dead 10 months later. What happened during that 10 months has had such a significant impact on my life, I doubt I can put it all into words.

I am the sixth of seven children. We were a close family; our father was a Baptist minister, and our mother, devoted to her children, was very proud that she had seven children. One of her favorite books and movies was *Cheaper by the Dozen,* by Frank Gilbreth, Jr. She taught us things early in life that have stayed with us. One of the biggest things she taught me is to love Jesus and the simple things in life. Each flower is beautiful to the beholder. Her favorites were violets and lilies of the valley, not expensive, but guess whose own garden has those flowers? (Were those really her favorite flowers? Or were they just the ones I remember picking for her? I don't really know.) So it is true—you do live on after death in those around you.

That's another thing I learned about my mother: I didn't really know her when she was alive. I was a child and I knew her as her child, for my needs. She knew me and what my needs were, but I never can imagine, even now, what she wanted or needed from me except to love her, and that was the easy part. That in itself was probably her best gift to me, to know how much she delighted in her children and her love for each of us.

I have learned much more about her since she passed on than I could have imagined. She has been gone now almost 34 years. It never ceases to amaze me that an old neighbor, church member, aunt, uncle, or cousin will start out the conversation by saying, "I was remembering your mother just the other day and.... " I love those stories. That is how I have learned about her as an adult. Sometimes those stories make me cry, but I still want to hear them! When the day is over and I am alone with my thoughts, I have those stories!

After Mother died, I never felt like a "victim," and I am so glad of that. But I did feel different. People around me told me I had to be special because God wouldn't allow a child to endure what we did if we were not equipped. I believed that and took it to heart. Sure, it was difficult and sometimes lonely. I cried myself to sleep every night for six months. That must have been so hard for my dad. Again, as a child, I never considered how much of a burden this must have been for him. I only cared about me.

No one could possibly ache more than I could! I remember hearing my father crying through the door of his friend's office after Mother's funeral. I had never heard my father cry before. I have never heard him cry since.

I am not certain what is the "best" way to give children the news regarding cancer. I believe the important thing is that you do it with love, and all else is irrelevant. When Mother became ill 34 years ago, they did not believe it was appropriate to tell children the "morbid" details, because they didn't want to destroy hope. I never believed my mother would die from breast cancer or anything else. It was a shock, but she had carefully laid out plans for others to step in and help with our needs and our father's need for support. She knew of a significant adult in each of our lives, and she contacted each of them without our knowing. She asked each of them to "take us under his wing" for a couple of special days to share important things about us that meant a lot to Mom. She even planned her own funeral so that Dad would not be burdened with too much amid all the stress.

I used to wonder why parents were reluctant to share important information with children of a terminally ill parent. I don't wonder anymore.

In May 1998, I was diagnosed with medullary carcinoma of the breast—the left breast, the same breast as my mother. I could not and did not tell my children. I did not want to interrupt their lives. Our daughter was busy with the pressure of finals in college, and our son was preparing for testing for his second-degree black belt. Mine was not a terminal diagnosis, but a devastating one. My husband told our children each individually as they came home from their day's activities. Of course, weighing on their minds was the potential that this disease might take me as it had their grandmother. I know it was in the back of their minds, as it had been in the back of my mind for years.

Cancer does not affect just the person with the disease, but that person's community: your immediate family, extended family, coworkers, friends, neighbors, etc. I think my mom was a very strong woman, and I felt strong as well. After the initial shock and surgeries, of course, I did talk with our children. I have cried with them.

They have busy lives. We have all returned to work and school and have tried to place cancer on the back burner. They know that none of us lives forever, but of course want their own family to live the longest! They also have hope. Their hope is Jesus Christ. And no matter what happens to our bodies here on Earth, they know that one day, we will live forever, wholly, healthy with Him.

It has been a comforting thought.

9

My Family Has Cancer

by Mary Robinson

My family has cancer—it just grows in *my* body. I work part time in sales, and I am a full-time mom. I have two wonderful boys: Chris, 11, and Cameron, 7.

I was diagnosed with breast cancer in 1992. In 1997, it was discovered that the cancer had metastasized to my bone and liver.

As I said, my family has cancer, it just grows in me. That is how we feel about cancer. It is a family issue.

I live with my heroes: Tom, my husband; Chris; and Cameron. My boys are very bright and offer much support. We hold family meetings and tell them first before we talk with other family members or friends and neighbors. We are honest and encourage lots of questions. Children will fantasize and fill in the blanks if they don't have the correct information. We read books from the library, visit the boys' classrooms at school, and try to keep their teachers informed. (The kids are very honest and accepting of everything—and they are fascinated with my bald head.)

My husband and I read to the boys at night. We lie down with them and talk. We give them five to 10 minutes of "ask any question" time. This has sparked many a conversation about treatment, school, death, fears, and hopes. We love this quiet time with our children, and we hope it will be something they treasure as much as we have. Cameron, when he was 6, told me one night he really preferred me bald. It warmed my heart.

When I was first diagnosed with breast cancer, Chris was 3 and Cameron was just 11 months old. I went through chemotherapy and radiation and went five years cancer-free. After I was diagnosed with metastatic cancer in the fall of 1997, we chose chemotherapy with a stem cell rescue transplant. It required at least a 21-day stay away from my family. It would be the first time I had been separated from Tom and the boys.

In preparation for this procedure, my husband and I discussed our fears and concerns. We both felt the biggest concern was anxiety about the unknown. Our goal was to have as much planned as possible so that while I was away, the boys would know who would be there for them, who would meet them off the bus, who would provide dinner each night—to try to maintain as normal a day-to-day schedule as possible. I made lists and calendars for every part of their day. I scheduled meals for almost every day, prepared a schedule for people to meet the boys off the bus, made an arrangement of play-dates up to a month in advance, compiled a list of friends' names with moms' names and phone numbers, wrote rules about snacks and bedtime rituals—all in an effort to assist the many caregivers (grandparents, friends, neighbors, etc.) who came to help my husband. In addition, we gave the boys journals to keep track of their feelings, and a list of things to do when they missed their mom. Neighborhood gifts of phone cards allowed us to talk every morning and night. Tom, with the help of family, friends, and neighbors, did it all with grace and style. I love him for all that he is: friend, lover, husband, father, driver, caregiver, and soul mate.

We experienced five months' success (cancer-free). Today, we are still battling cancer in my liver.

I am still very healthy except for the cancer. I am fortunate to be able to run three to five miles at least five days a week and live a normal active lifestyle. We have a saying in my family: We don't concentrate on "Am I going to die from this cancer?" but rather, "How can we learn to live with this cancer?"

My 11-year-old son Chris once said a very wise thing during a family meeting. In our attempt to explain chronic illness to our boys, we were talking about my starting treatment again and how it will be a way of life. We said we were not sure how much time we would have between each new treatment. Chris stopped us and said, "Let's not talk about the next time, Mom and Dad, let's concentrate on right now." How beautifully put, Chris. Thank you.

Yesterday is the past. Tomorrow is the future. Today is the present, and that's why we call it a gift.

My name is Christopher.

My mom's name is Mary, and she has cancer. I was 4 when I learned that my mom had cancer. Now I am 11.

Of course, at the time I was 4, I did not think much of it until I learned more about it. But I knew my mom would always be there.

I knew mostly everything because we talked about it a lot. What helped me most was focusing on the positive things and not the negative. God is always up there looking down on us and protecting us—and my mom.

My mom's cancer has recurred, and obviously the thing to

do is do what she did last time because it worked pretty well. My advice to other kids when someone in your family has cancer is to ask a lot of questions because you need to know what is going on.

My advice to parents is to ask your kids if they have any questions, and try to answer them the best way you can. And to tell your kids things you want them to know because if kids do not know what's going on, then they will probably be even more scared than they already are.

And overall, be happy, because you are the same person you always were. Just a little more special.

My name is Cameron.

My mom has breast cancer. I was a baby when my mom first had cancer. I really liked to rub her bald head when I was little. Now I am 7.

Cancer makes me feel bad because it just does. I think it might make people die.

The letters my mom wrote from the hospital in Chicago made me feel better. I felt better when my dad's countdown calendar was at one day after my mom was in the hospital for 20 days.

I liked it when Dad said Mom was going to be okay. And after the 21 days, I loved it when my mom came home.

10
Ready to Enter Chemotherapy

by Fred

Here is our story. I was diagnosed with Gleason 7 Stage D2 metastatic bulky prostate cancer at the age of 55 in 1997, after my wife and I returned from Thailand, when our daughter was 11 and son had just turned 15. We had very little savings. Complicating the family survival issue was that my wife spoke faltering English.

Hormone ablation treatment failed after only eight months, but I was able to buy some six months of stabilized PSA (an indicator of cancer growth) by getting Nizoral from Mexico. That eventually failed. I am currently getting ready to enter chemotherapy as the cancer has metastasized to the bone, and lymph disruption has caused genital lymphedema. Almost no free trial protocols are running for prostate cancer patients, and there are none in our area.

My son is now 16 and my daughter will soon to turn 13. Within nine months of my diagnosis, my wife took a minimum-wage factory job doing cleaning with industrial solvents and other risky tasks. She continues to hold the job. As her skills, including English, improve, we hope she will become prepared to obtain a more satisfying and stable job. As much as our budget would allow, we immediately began taking out high-priced "no medical questions asked" term life insurance policies for me because they will pay off for a death due to illness, but only after two years. As the two-year policy anniversary approaches, we know that we will have at least some benefits paid when I die.

My son was able to find a summer job when he was only 15. Now in school, he continues to work for the same company one day a week. He had to drop his sports activities in order to keep his grades up. My wife takes free ESL (English as a Second Language) classes twice a week. My son is taking accounting in school and now has a driver's license and a credit card. My daughter studies consumer math in middle school and is devoted to the family cat. I find some miscellaneous income when I am up to it by buying, fixing, and reselling old computers at swap meets.

I give intensive backup and support to my wife and children, as they will need to have a stable routine in order to hold together as a family when I am gone. I am preplanning a cremation with a simple service. We really carry on as if things are normal except that one of us, Dad, is seriously sick. We are fearful, of course, of the day the sickness turns to absence, and sometimes my mind wonders how well each of the three will be able to take the loss. I realize each will be strongly affected in his or her own way, and they all will carry on bravely as people always have. They will become a tighter trio, and school friends and neighbors will help by accommodating some of the adjustments they will be struggling at first to make.

We don't panic. We try to make steady progress toward preparing for the inevitable. Since the diagnosis, we are all more pleasant, patient, and loving with each other and that has been our strength for dealing with each step along the way. We cultivate a toughness, too—one that unfortunately brings early cynicism and maturity.

We do not see ourselves as a special case. We know that the cycle of life is one that we, like everyone else, participate in. I am content with my life's course, and our family believes that human beings and life are good.

11
Speaking With the Angels

by John Gaffney

I have to start with a dream. My dream of the white wolf. It happened on June 19, 2000, the night before my son, Aidan, was born. In the dream I was walking through a wide open field, bordered by thick briar bushes. I wandered into the briar bushes and sat down, hiding in them for some unknown reason. I heard a rustling behind me. Something big, I thought. A huge white wolf approached through the brush. I wasn't scared. It stopped close to me and sat down, then laid down. Then I woke up. The day and the dream were quickly absorbed in the joy and drama of Aidan's birth.

Fast forward. It's four years later, April 4, 2004. If you were Aidan or his nine-year-old sister, Annelise, here's what you saw. Your grandparents were here from Croatia to help take care of you while your mother shuttled to Middlesex Hospital for the past 35 days. Your father has been very sick and the constant flow of family members combined with his absence has given you the sense that something has gone very wrong. At 2:00 p.m. on that day your mother walked through the door with a man that looked like your father, but his complexion was very gray. He was very skinny, very slow and very bald.

Here's what I saw that day. After a 35-day bout with massive chemotherapy to combat Acute Promylocetic Myeloid Leukemia (APML), complete with trips to ICU and CCU, I was coming home to the two reasons that inspired me to fight through every one of those 35 days: My kids. But when I walked in the door that day and reached to pick up Aidan he said, "That's not my Daddy." He hid behind his grandfather. Probably a good thing because I wasn't strong enough to pick him up. I went upstairs to where Annelise, who had been a pretty cool customer when she visited me in the hospital a week before, was hysterically crying. I hugged her. "It's okay now," I said. "I'm home."

I was home, but it wasn't okay. It was the first day of a mysterious, emotional, painful and ultimately transcendent journey for me and my family. There was plenty more chemo to be dealt my way, plenty of drama including another hospital stay in July. But what I realized is that cancer for kids is a journey marked by angels. Dark angels sometimes, messenger angels other times, but angels nonetheless. Cancer gave my kids an opportunity to learn about complex emotions like grief, unexplainable sadness and fear. It also taught them to rely on other people for help with those emotions.

As I look back over the two years of my APML treatment, it's the transcendent moments with my kids that stand out among all the needles and nausea. They stand taller than the physical and emotional struggles. Those moments actually started with the white wolf. About a week after I got home from the hospital, my wife gave Aidan a book for me to read to him. She had ordered it to help the kids relate to my struggle. It was called *Henry and the White Wolf*. Henry was a young groundhog who was sick. His mother had always taught him to stay away from the lair of the white wolf, but in this story, Henry's sickness can only be cured by a potion possessed by the wolf. The white wolf tells Henry that the potion will make him much sicker and cause him to lose all his fur. But it will eventually return him to health. All of this comes to pass in the story, and Henry is no longer afraid of the white wolf. I go back to that dream I had the night before Aidan was born. For me the briars were the cancer; the white wolf the cure. Aidan was the messenger.

There were a few more moments with Aidan that I am still amazed by. For as early as he could talk, Aidan has always spoken with great confidence about his experience as an angel. He told me many times that he was an angel before he "went into Mommy's tummy." That connection took on new meaning in early December of 2005. I received a positive result from one of my blood tests. Suddenly my miraculous recovery was being stained by phrases like "arsenic trioxide" and "stem cell transplant." The pressure was intense. We went away to Stockbridge, Massachusetts, during the first weekend in December. Stockbridge is where Norman Rockwell lived and worked. They have a Christmas festival every year, which the kids didn't seem to care as much about as the indoor pool at the hotel where we stayed. One afternoon, I was sitting by the pool looking out of the window at the snow falling. I was obsessed with the results of the blood test and fearful of my future. Aidan knew nothing about the blood test. But as I was sitting that day in my fear, Aidan said: "Daddy, did you know that when I was an angel, I picked this family to come to because I knew you had leukemia. I'm here to help you with your leukemia."

Stunned, I said the first thing that came to my mind. "Is it going to kill me?"

"No," he said. "But you're going to have to go to the doctor a lot."

A month later, a definitive bone marrow test showed my blood test to be a false positive. No stem cell transplant. Just seven months more of going to the doctor a lot.

Annelise's transformation was helped immensely by The Children's Treehouse Foundation and their support program, CLIMB (Children's Lives Include Moments of Bravery). She went to the first support group for kids at Middlesex Hospital's cancer center in October 2005. On the ride up to the first meeting, I asked her why she was crying so much the day I came home from the hospital. She didn't know. Six weeks later she had a chance to explore all the emotions that came with this dark angel of cancer. She had a chance to meet other kids whose parents and grandparents had been through worse. She learned to be comfortable with the words "sad" and "fear." She even connected with the concept of emotion.

After we walked in that same door in December 2005, and after The Children's Treehouse CLIMB workshops were over, I again asked Annelise why she was crying that day when I first came home from the hospital. "I was sad, Daddy," she said. "You know sometimes all these feelings just come at you at the same time."

Time. Time the healer. Time the avenger. Time is what kids can teach you about. We think we're teaching them how to deal with cancer, but there are higher forces at work. Ask my kids. Now they'll tell you.

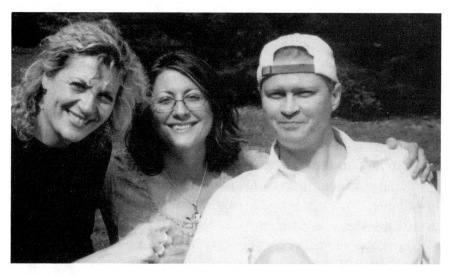

John Gaffney, six weeks after major chemotherapy treatment and two days before returning to the hospital with an E. coli infection and 104 degree fever, with wife Lillian, center, and family friend Renee, left.

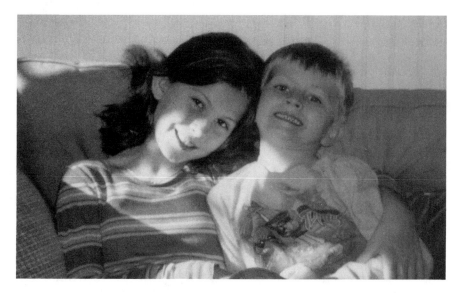

Annelise, left, and Aidan, right.

12

I Am Ashamed

by Audrey Rankin

I am ashamed. When I was diagnosed with chondrosarcoma bone cancer, it was devastating. I could not bring myself to tell my two children. No one should have to tell her children that she has cancer. They found out from their cousin. My daughter is still very, very hurt from this. I will always feel bad about it. I wasn't strong and just didn't have the guts to tell them. My son was 9 at the time and didn't even want to be in the same room with me. Didn't even want to be near me.

Once they knew, I always let them know what was going on. I brought them along with me for my appointments at the Mayo Clinic in Minnesota. They got to meet the doctor, which put them somewhat at ease. They saw what my day was like, going through testing, etc. My daughter and mother were with me when I finally got my body cast off. My son enjoys going to Mayo with me. It's a great adventure, from staying in a hotel that has a swimming pool to all the different people we see. It's a learning experience all the way around.

What works is involvement. Not keeping anything from them. Trying to put their mind at ease.

What didn't work was letting my anxiety show. I feel like I could crack up. I still have not found a way to let my stress out. I have no peace. Keeping something important from them only makes it worse for them. If it's bad news or great news, they have to know and be included.

Finding out I had cancer April 1, 1996, I should have told them then—and that's no fooling! The shock of it. Not understanding what was in store for myself, I could not even begin to tell them what was going to happen. I wanted to be strong, and I wanted my children to hear the cancer news from me. I couldn't bring myself to tell them. I feel I let them down big time! I was weak.

We went to the March for Cancer in September 1998, in Washington, D.C. My husband, Pat; the kids, Ashley and Josh; and me! It was our first family trip. First time on an airplane. First time ever doing anything like this. It was such a moving experience for all of us. It was incredible. We saw that so many people are touched by cancer—young and old alike. That experience really pulled us together in more ways than one.

Now, I belong to a support group. It helps us all to stay strong.

From daughter Ashley:

I was shocked. I didn't know how to react when I was told. I would have liked to know what exactly was going to happen, and to know that she was going to be okay.

And from son Josh:

I didn't know what was going on. I wanted to know would my mom be okay. My sister told me about it.

13
Something Is Wrong!

by Teresa Beck

Even though very young children don't understand what is going on, they do understand one thing: *Something is wrong!*

I was diagnosed with a rare form of vulva cancer about two weeks before my 38th birthday. It was about three months before my son Matthew's third birthday. My husband and I were devastated. The only folks we had known with cancer had both died within months of diagnosis. Our initial diagnosis led us to believe the same would happen to me. It turned out, though, that the doctors felt they caught it at stage one; nine months later, I am healthy and cancer-free. It required surgery with no radiation or chemotherapy.

Despite the ease of the cure, it was very traumatic for all of us. I was still nursing Matthew, and I decided I needed to wean him before the surgery. I did this two weeks before the surgery, hoping that he would not associate the weaning with the surgery or hospital stay. I weaned him abruptly, telling him that my "mum-mums" were sick and had no more milk. Since he was close to weaning himself, he did well except for bedtime. After about five days, he seemed okay with the new set of rules. It was an extremely difficult time for both of us. I felt guilty, like I was betraying him. I was taking away his security at a time when I felt he/we needed it the most.

Matthew was still very attached to me. We were still having separation problems each morning at school. He also didn't

adapt well to change. I knew this was going to be a very difficult time for him.

My parents stayed with us for several days after the diagnosis, then came back for five weeks for the surgery and
recovery. This kept Matthew entertained, although he was
showing signs of stress (an increase in attachment issues). I
explained that my boo-boo was back and I needed to go to the
hospital for the doctors to make it go away.

Prior to my going to the hospital, I checked children's
books out of the library about going to the hospital. I
explained to Matthew I would be going for a few days. I had to
go only because doctors had special tools there that they did-
n't have at their offices. I pointed out all the things in the hospital I thought he would see... the beds on wheels, the beds
that go up and down, IV bottles, oxygen tanks, etc.

Prior to the surgery, I asked the daycare center not to move
him to the 3-year-old room (he was about to moved when I
found out about the cancer). They obliged and left him in the
classroom he was comfortable in. I knew his attachment to
his teacher there would help him.

During the hospital stay, my parents kept Matthew busy.
When I left the hospital after four days, he knew every elevator in the building and where it went. He seemed afraid to
come into my hospital room, afraid of me, and very worried.
No amount of reassurance seemed to help him. My parents
held him a lot. (My husband was too upset to deal well with
Matthew at the time.)

I tried to make the hospital trip fun by pointing out all the
things he had seen in his books about hospitals. When we
went for a walk at the hospital, I pointed out all the things we
saw in the books. I had trouble explaining the catheter and

urine bag. They weren't in the books, and they seemed to scare him. I did remember that his favorite movie, *Apollo 13*, had a urine bag in it, so I called it my astronaut bag. He thought that was neat. He got a new toy each day, so that provided some diversion.

Once we got home, he curled up in bed with me. He spent the first weekend there, day and night. We just talked and watched TV. After that, it was obvious he expected things to be back to normal— and they weren't. It was about three weeks before I could get up and around with any ease. His attachment was even more pronounced. He had regressed in potty training, going from almost trained to wanting to wear diapers and have me change him.

After about two days of my mother's changing the dressing on the drain hole in my abdomen, she called Matthew to watch. We were undecided as to whether this would help or scare him more. It actually was a turning point in his ability to handle the situation.

He saw this small incision, only about a quarter of an inch long and heard my mother tell me how clean it looked and how it was healing well. You could see the curiosity and relief on his face. He saw his foe, and it was manageable.

He still asks about my "cancer boo-boo." It is obvious he is concerned and doesn't fully understand it. Sometimes, when he hears about someone else being sick or dying, he asks about my boo-boo. I assure him it is gone and he doesn't have to worry about me. He seems to feel better and drops the subject as quickly as it came up.

It took about five months after the surgery before he potty trained himself again. He also still tells me he misses having "mum-mum" and asks if my mum-mums are okay and are they making milk again. Again, I talk to him about it. Talking seems to help him.

In summary, the things I think helped:

- We told him about the "boo-boo," giving it a name. We talked about it whenever he wanted, trying to address the things we knew would concern him (separation, changing of routine, not understanding Mommy being "hurt").

- We got books about hospitals. We tried to make a game out of looking for all the things we had read about.

- He got a new toy each day I was in the hospital.

- We used diversion. My parents did a great job of entertaining him while I was in the hospital and recovering.

- My parents also got him out of the house when my husband and I were having a particularly rough time coping.

- I tried to keep the daycare environment and daily routine as stable as possible.

- I kept assuring him all would be okay. (Of course, I realize I was lucky that actually was the case.)

- My son is very verbal for a 3-year-old. I let him talk, ask questions, etc. I answered everything I could, trying to anticipate and address his fears. I tried to tell him everything that would happen before it occurred so that he would have no surprises to scare him.

- I held him as much as possible; indulging his dependency needs and giving him the freedom to regress in his behavior seemed to help. The talking, holding, reassurance, and allowing regressions in behavior seemed to be what he needed most.

14
Goompa Has an Owie

by Sue Browne

SON: *Why does Goompa have an owie? Did he fall down, or did somebody hit him? I want to see him. Mommy, can I?*

MOM: *We can't see Grandpa because he is in the hospital. He and Grandma live far away. Remember when we went on the airplane to see him at his new house?*

SON: *So, let's go on an airplane, go seeyum, 'kay?*

MOM: *We don't have enough money, sweetie.*

SON: *But I have some more money in my piggy bank. I want to give Goompa a hug-kiss.*

MOM: *We'll go see him soon.*

SON: *All right!*

It is impossible to explain cancer to a 4-year-old. He loves his grandpa so much that it breaks our hearts to explain how sick Grandpa is now. I think that just leaving it at, "He's real sick," is the best explanation. Also, when we talk to him about Grandpa, and we get a tear or two in our eyes, we don't try to hide it. He needs to see our sadness, but he also needs to hear us talk very positively and lovingly about Grandpa. It is a matter of balance.

We are going to make a video of Grandpa talking to all his

grandkids. He'll likely have some of that good ole Grandpa advice saturated in wisdom and love. We hope that when the memories fade of what their grandpa looks and sounds like, they can look at their video and feel so much love and feel so special that it will be hard to ignore. This is one way of turning cancer into a gift.

15
I Love Life!

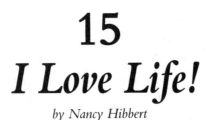

by Nancy Hibbert

At age 42, I was diagnosed with breast cancer. The diagnosis came a week before my husband, our 6-year-old daughter, Andrea, and I were to go to Hawaii for spring break. This vacation was special to Andrea since she was scheduled to "swim with the dolphins."

I had the dual task of explaining that the vacation was to be postponed, and that Mommy needed to see some doctors. She was disappointed about the trip, yet not particularly concerned that I needed medical help.

I did not tell my daughter that I had breast cancer. I did not use the word cancer at all, because in many contexts it has such a "fatal" component. Our communication centered on what she might notice about my health from an outward appearance, especially the loss of hair. We turned my hair loss into a celebration—she would be the only kindergartner with a "bald mom." She suggested a green wig! She quickly told all the other kids in kindergarten that I was going to be bald. She felt special and unique. Eventually, all the kindergartners wanted to see my bald head and touch it. The boys with short crew cuts thought it was outrageously funny that they had more hair than I did.

Another strategy that we employed was to have Andrea "sleep over" with relatives for the first few days of the chemotherapy. She thought it was a treat, and I didn't have to worry about her seeing me suffering from side effects.

It wasn't until we decided to participate in the Race for the Cure that we talked about my illness being breast cancer. Now, she is alert to the words and always notifies me of any TV or newspaper story about breast cancer. She "knows" that by the time she grows up, there will be a vaccine. My daughter never feared my cancer, and it allowed us to use our energy on loving, having fun, and making memories.

I have had a great team, including a strong network of breast cancer survivors who shared their stories, tips, and practical life insights. I've enjoyed caring and compassionate words from my peers, predominantly men in the engineering and construction trades. Wonderful health-care givers treated me as if I were their first and only patient. An employer gave unconditional support. My husband rallied to do all the child care and house chores. This great team allowed me to maintain a positive outlook.

The diagnosis starts a whirlwind of decisions and appointments, and often the children are "left out." What to say, how to say it, and what is age-appropriate are all so very important considerations.

Often the parents don't ever want to share the news. My father died from Hodgkin's disease when I was 15, and my parents never told me how serious the illness was, so I never got the chance to really say good-bye.

I am convinced that I am cancer free, and never once considered my cancer to be life threatening. I love life!

16
Baldy Head...Hair Head

by Heller Bates

On April 14, 1997, I was diagnosed with breast cancer. Our daughter, Madilyn, was invited to go to a birthday party for her cousin, who was turning 3, on the same day I received the devastating news. We went to the birthday party anyway, and nobody (including Madi) knew what we had just found out. I should have received an Academy Award that day; Madi had a great time, and it would not have been fair for her to miss that party.

I had been working in sales for the past 14 years for the same company, and I had decided that it was time to give my notice and stay home and raise our child. I had felt the lump before I gave my notice, but I never really thought it could be cancer. If I had known my summer with my child would turn into my summer with chemotherapy, I would not have resigned. It gave me entirely too much time to think.

On May 2, 1997, I underwent a lumpectomy. The surgeon took 29 lymph nodes; all were cancerous. I was to go through four rounds of chemotherapy and then have a bone marrow transplant. At this point, Madi (who turned 3 on July 3, 1997) didn't know what was going on, so one day I sat down to have a talk with her. I told her that I was sick and was going to get sicker before I could get better. I also told her I was going to lose all my hair from the medicine they were going to give me, and wouldn't that be silly. She accepted everything because I was very open with her and let her know what to expect, so when the time came, she knew. I also had a Groshong catheter put in my chest, so when I got home from having that done, I showed it to her. When I had to clean it, she would help me put the dressing on it. Instead of it frightening her, she felt she was helping to make me better.

On August 18, 1997, I went into the hospital for a stem cell transplant. I was given the option of doing it as an outpatient or in the hospital. I opted for the hospital so Madi would not have to see me really sick. I'm very glad that I chose that, because I had a few days when I wouldn't let her come see me. I think seeing me that sick would have frightened her. I know it scared me. Other than that time, my husband brought her almost every day. I would try to make it fun for her by playing with the cool hospital bed or just playing. The nurses were wonderful and made Madi feel very special.

When I came home from the hospital, it took at least a month to start feeling any better. I had been in the hospital for 24 days and now that I was home, I think Madi thought I should be all better. This was the worst time for her because I had no energy, and she didn't understand why and kept wondering when I was going to get better. I didn't have an answer for her because I was wondering the same thing. It did help when people would come take her to play with their children, or she would go to daycare. Finally, I started feeling better so I would spend most of my energy on Madi, and we grew closer.

The thing Madi and I remember about that time is Madi's patting me on the head and saying, "Baldy head, baldy head." (Now she pats me on the head and says, "Hair head, hair head.") We also joked that since Halloween was just around the corner, I could go as Uncle Fester from the Addams Family.

I handled the cancer and Madi with honesty and tried not to lose my sense of humor. I was one year out of the hospital on August 26, 1998, and we celebrated with friends who made me a birthday cake. I'm not sure that, at 4 years old, Madi really understood, but she does understand that she has her Mommy back, healthy and strong. We talk about the hospital and my walking around with my IV pole, but it's less frequent now. At least she knows she can always talk about it and, I hope, talk about it when I'm an old woman!

17

Children: The Forgotten Part of Cancer

by Wendy Lindstrom, R.N.

I have been caring for cancer patients since I was 2 years old. How is this possible? you might ask.

I'm now an oncology nurse, but the first cancer patient I cared for was my dad. He was diagnosed with non-Hodgkin's lymphoma when I was 2, and the cancer recurred about six years later. Two months after we celebrated his 40th birthday, my father died. I was 10 years old.

My mother told me he had noticed a lump in his groin while taking a shower, shortly before a family camping trip. He went to see his doctor and soon began treatment. Because I was so young when my father was diagnosed, nothing seemed out of the ordinary. Looking back, one of my few memories of his first treatment was a trip to the hospital. My dad was too sick to drive himself home from outpatient treatment, so my mother and I went to the hospital to pick him up.

About six years later, my dad's cancer recurred. Although I didn't know he had cancer, let alone a recurrence, I definitely noticed the changes in our household. I remember the blue and purple marks on my father's neck and chest (from radiation treatments), several trips to the local pharmacy, and bottles of medication always in the house. I can still recall my father's pale skin every time he needed a blood transfusion, his Hickman catheter, his sunken eyes and thin body (which once had a round belly), and his disappearing light blonde hair.

My dad did not want to tell my sister or me that he had cancer. (My mother has since explained his silence on the subject.) He had beaten this disease once, and he was determined to do so again.

While cancer was not discussed at home, my parents made sure we shared good times during my dad's illness. We spent two weeks in Scandinavia, visiting distant relatives in Sweden and traveling the region. My sister joined us for a few days while she traveled a more extensive itinerary with my grandmother, my father's mother. It was the last summer vacation we took together. Even then my father didn't look well. He was fatigued, pale, thin, and had lost a lot of his hair.

Later, he was too sick to make it down five stairs during our last Christmas together. We were able to get him into a wheelchair and wheel him to the top of the staircase while my sister, mother, and I opened presents below, beside our family Christmas tree. I didn't know what was going on, but I knew something wasn't right. I had chickenpox after that Christmas (a month before he died), so we were both at home, taking care of each other. We wrapped homemade candy and watched TV while he rested in bed.

One moment I won't forget was when he was changing the dressing on his Hickman catheter. I watched as blood came spurting out of the catheter; this was before one-way valves were introduced. At first we were frightened, but soon we were giggling because the blood almost hit the ceiling.

I don't think I truly knew he was not going to get better until a few weeks before my father died. My mother, sister, and I were at the hospital when my mother asked my father where he wanted to be buried. My mom apologized for scaring my sister and me, but she said she needed to ask my father this important question. He was in pain and almost incoherent, but he did know he wanted to be buried next to his father in Connecticut.

I will never forget the moment when I learned my father had died. While the death of a loved one is never forgotten, I particularly remember it because it came as such a shock. It was a late Monday afternoon, and my sister and I were home from school. We were in our living room doing our homework and watching TV when the phone rang. My sister answered the phone in the kitchen, in plain view of the living room. She spoke only briefly before she screamed, "Daddy's dead!" I ran in disbelief and horror up to my room, screaming at the top of my lungs, "No!" I curled up in a ball on the floor and started punching my bed. My sister ran after me and held me as we cried together. It was a close family friend who had called. He wanted to know how my sister and I were doing, but my mother had not yet come home from the hospital to tell us about our father.

I didn't understand death. I had been waiting for my mother to come home and take me to the hospital to see my dad. I couldn't wait to see him. I was hurrying to finish my homework so I would be ready to go when my mother got home. Everything was supposed to be getting better. It was Monday. I had just seen him on Saturday. My mother had said he was doing better over the weekend. Suddenly he was gone.

After my dad died, it was clear no one knew what to say beyond the words "I'm sorry." My family's friends weren't sure how I would react. I was excused from everything. My teacher told my class what had happened. On my first day back to school, my best friend told me the teacher said I could get up and leave class at any time, without asking for permission. I remember thinking that was an odd thing to say. At the funeral, my piano teacher told me I was excused from piano practice. I loved playing the piano and my dad always listened to me play, so I did not want to stop practicing. I met with the school psychologist a few times, but she worked primarily with students who had learning disabilities. She told my mother about a few books written for children about grief and loss. While it was helpful to read stories about other children going through similar situations, it still didn't answer my question: Why did my dad die?

After my father's death, even though I didn't feel close to my mother, I realized she was the only parent I had left and I was afraid of losing her. Losing my dad had been so unexpected; what was going to stop my mother from being taken away from me? My mother soon started a new job and had a different schedule every day. I was always nervous from the time I got home from school until she returned safely from work. If she was late getting home because she stopped at the grocery store to pick up dinner, I panicked. I was afraid she had been hurt in a car accident somewhere and that was why she wasn't home on time.

We didn't talk much about it, but our family continued to experience changes as a result of my father's death. These changes were difficult to deal with. We took our first family vacation without my dad, and my mom changed careers to make more money. I remember my mom looking at me as she cried and said it was hard for her, too. I just kept thinking, "But you're the mom. You're supposed to know what to do and how to fix things." She didn't. She started dating about six months after my father's death. She dated the same man for about five years, and at one time they almost bought a house together. It was very obvious to me that my mother was trying to get her life back together. She had a new man in her life and a new career. I also thought it was obvious that having children just didn't fit into her "new life."

When I was in junior high school, my sister and I were referred to a school counselor to participate in grief groups. One group was for high school students and one for junior high students, so my sister and I were not in the same group. While I am glad they were trying to address the issue and help us work through our feelings, school was not the right place to do it. It was very difficult to spend 47 minutes talking about death, grief, and loss, then stop the discussion when the bell rang and return to class to concentrate on algebra. The group did bring me a new friend, Sabrina. She was in one of my classes, but we didn't know we both had lost our fathers. Sabrina's father had a heart attack and died during a family vacation. The counselor often said how difficult it must have been for her because her father's death was so sudden and unexpected. I kept thinking to myself, "How many kids expect their parents to die?" I certainly didn't. I hadn't even known my dad had cancer or what cancer was. I didn't consider hospitalization very serious. I knew babies were born in hospitals, and they were fine. I got stitches in the emergency room one time, and I was fine. My dad went to the hospital sometimes for treatments, but he always came home.

After about a semester, Sabrina and I both decided we couldn't go to any more of the grief sessions. We found them too depressing. The room was dark; it was often full of dead silence because kids didn't want to talk and get upset and then go back to classes. My mother could see that I was still having trouble. She asked if I wanted to see a therapist, but at the time I thought only crazy people went to therapists. I didn't understand that this was a normal thing to do after experiencing the death of a parent.

My sister is four years older than I am, so she was 14 when my father died. As a typical teenager, she was spending more and more time with her friends. She was just starting to date and was developing a new support system among her friends. I think her age, her friends, and the fact that she was closer to my mother helped her deal with my father's death. A year after his death, she was driving to after-school activities and working. It wasn't long before she was off to college.

All my feelings and unresolved grief caught up with me one day. I had not completed an assignment on time, so my teacher reprimanded me. She was so threatening it made me angry. After class, I was walking down the main hallway when I saw a friend and burst into tears. I couldn't handle things anymore. I couldn't handle my mother anymore. Something had to change.

I started seeing the school counselor again, this time in one-on-one sessions instead of a group. Again, it was hard to talk about feelings and then return to class. Sometimes I would be late to the next class because I just couldn't go back after being so upset. The school counselor would try to calm me down and handed me a few tissues, but that just didn't cut it. I was frustrated that we were just talking about feelings. I wanted to know how to fix things and make things better so I wouldn't feel like this anymore. Despite arguments with my mother and 20-page letters I wrote her to express my feelings, my relationship with her did not change for many years. I looked for support elsewhere. I grew closer with friends from school and their families. After high school, I wanted to get as far away from home as possible. My mother said I could go to college anywhere as long as it was on the East Coast. I went as far away as possible—to Florida.

In Florida I started volunteering at the university's hospital. I started out in physical therapy and the newborn nursery but quickly found my way to the pediatric oncology and bone-marrow transplant units. I volunteered for the American Cancer Society and decided to major in health education. Before I graduated, I decided to attend nursing school because I wanted to be an oncology nurse.

I realized I love working with cancer patients and their families. And I've learned how critically important it is to have open communications.

A diagnosis of cancer changes a family forever. Figuring out what's for dinner or what to do during the upcoming weekend are suddenly less important questions. Family and personal values are questioned, and priorities are tested. As an oncology nurse, I have seen old, unsettled feelings and arguments resurface during a family's struggle with cancer. Often family members must revisit and sort out old, unre-solved feelings before they can start to battle cancer as a family.

Children are often the forgotten part of cancer. I have seen this as a nurse and as a child of a cancer patient. It's not because people forget about the children. It's because no one knows what to say or how to help them. I find it truly ironic that out of all the health-care professionals who cared for my dad, the only one I remember is the social worker from my father's inpatient oncology unit. No doubt this is because she always took the time to talk with my family and always included my sister and me.

During childhood and adolescence, coping skills are still

developing. This is why talking to children about cancer is essential. The information should be in small doses, in words they can understand. Although it is important to try to maintain a "normal" schedule and lifestyle for children, they also need to be included in the more serious discussions. Remember that children look to their parents for information and understanding. Talking with children shows them that their parents are there for support. It also encourages kids to talk about their problems and their feelings. When parents choose to hide information, children do not feel a part of the family unit that is fighting cancer. If children are not given information, they may seek it by eavesdropping on adults' conversations, or they may fill in the gaps with their imagination.

Although some people tell me my work must be depressing, it isn't. I enjoy being with patients and their families, educating them about cancer, and caring for them. After dealing with cancer in my family, I know first-hand that answering a family's questions and being there for them during a difficult time is what they need. To my surprise, the most common question from my patients in an inpatient hospital unit is, "Do you like what you do?" I always reply, "I could never be an operating room or an emergency room nurse, but oncology nursing—I can't imagine doing anything else."

18
Cool, Mom!

by Luanne Dossett

I am a full-time mom and kindergarten teacher, and I am married to Jim and have two children. I was diagnosed with breast cancer three years ago at the age of 40. My son, Kylor, was 9 and in third grade. My daughter, Sharayah, was 6 and in kindergarten. My husband was teaching physical education, and I was working as a paraprofessional in the same school that my kids attended.

I received a phone call while at work and was shocked to hear the results of my biopsy. The first thing that entered my mind was my kids. I knew I would do whatever I could to watch my kids grow up. I immediately told my husband, as the news spread among the staff. If I had not found out at school, I would not have told anybody quite so soon, but as it turned out, we had an instant support group. Talking about it right away was the best medicine that could be prescribed. That afternoon, I calmly told my children about my diagnosis. I was honest with them but optimistic about my future. Sharayah cried at first, but with calm reassurance from Jim and me, she and Kylor handled the news very well. Kids are going to react like those around them, so it is important to plan what you are going to say.

Prior to my mastectomy, I explained the procedure to my kids and showed them pictures so they knew what to expect. My daughter was very interested and accompanied me to subsequent doctor appointments.

I also went through six treatments of chemotherapy. During that time, it helped me to continue working, exercising, and attending our kids' activities. When we were able to maintain our normal schedule, it helped our kids as well. We had a lot of support from the school staff, community members, church, friends, and family.

One of the most difficult events I experienced was losing my hair. One day, after buzzing my son's hair, I locked myself in the bathroom and buzzed my own. After I shed tears with my daughter and my husband, my son walked in and said, "Cool, Mom!" That relieved the tension and was a big relief to me. Because I had planned to wear scarves and hats, the next day was declared Hat Day at school for staff and students.

Later that summer, between treatments, I interviewed for and accepted another teaching job. That was an exciting time for my whole family. It was good for them to see that even when life is difficult, good things can still happen—a powerful example for their future.

Kids are very resilient. Because we were honest, maintained a positive attitude, and felt confident that we could get through this challenge, the kids reacted with the same level of courage and confidence.

My husband was a saint during this experience. Jim was very supportive and continues to be so. He is a great role model for our children. Through family, friends, community, and prayer, we made it. I thank God for every day that I have the opportunity to watch my children grow.

My name is Kylor. *I am 12 years old and in the sixth grade. I remember coming home from a friend's house and finding my mom, dad, and sister in the bathroom* *shaving my mom's hair off. I was shocked, but I thought it was cool because I had my head shaved. I felt sorry for my mom.*

All the things our friends—like Mrs. Baumgartner, one of my second grade teachers—did, like bring good food and give us support, helped us a lot.

My name is Sharayah, *and I am 9 years old. I was 6 when I found out my mom had breast cancer. I cried because I was scared. I had a friend who had a mom who lost her hair and that helped. I felt I had to help my mom, so I went with her to her doctor appointments. If your mom or dad has cancer, it helps to talk to a friend. Now, it's back to normal and I'm glad.*

19
Yes, Mom, I'm Scared

by Georgia Mucilli, R.N.

My husband Steve had just driven off, when I removed my pajama top and my thumb hit a lump in my breast. Wow! That set me back! I knew that lump was not present when I checked my breast the previous month. I had my annual checkup the month before, and my gynecologist hadn't found it either. Being a surgical nurse, I had helped remove cancer from many patients. This lump was so hard and different from the fibrocystic mass I had. I was scared to death. My family history predisposed me to breast cancer, as my mother had breast cancer 28 years prior. The only thing holding me together was the fact that Mom is still here to tell about it.

Things moved quickly, which I felt was necessary. I was in my internist's office the same afternoon. He could not aspirate it. On Tuesday of the next week, I had a mammogram showing a solitary mass, and the next day the radiologist biopsied it under ultrasound. I had lobular breast cancer. The good news was the mass was small.

Steve had taken my 11-year-old daughter Veronica to the airport that morning. She had left for a 10-day trip with my girlfriend and her family. This gave me time to deal with the biopsy and diagnosis without facing Veronica each day. I turned to my mother and asked her what to say. Mom advised, gently, with honesty, stress the positives, and remind her that Grandma had cancer and is still with us.

Looking back, the first time Mom had cancer, I was 7. She

didn't tell us it was malignant colon polyps, but that she was facing a very big surgery and would be in the hospital three weeks. I knew it was serious by the look on her face and her gentle tears. I had a feeling she might not be with me always, but the fact that she kept trying kept me going.

Mom beat the colon cancer, but she still has changes in her routine that she deals with daily. Her spirit always kept me going. Then, when I was 18, Mom found the breast lump. Wham, that hit me like a punch! She discussed the surgery and risks honestly, and stressed it was small, which was in her favor. After the surgeon reported he had removed all of the tumor with a radical mastectomy and there was no cancer in the lymph nodes, something inside told me that Mom was going to be okay. Honestly, I knew there was a chance I'd have to help Dad raise my four siblings, but Mom had made me capable. Mom had also taught us to pray, and pray we did!

I told Veronica the second day she was home. Her reaction was totally unexpected. I barely got "breast cancer" out of my mouth when she started crying hysterically. "I don't want you to die!" I asked her where she had heard that people always die from breast cancer, because today there are many sur-vivors. "Last night on TV, Mom, I saw a lady dying from breast cancer." TV! She had watched only 15 minutes before bed. TV—just one of the many reasons our kids know so much more than I did 40 years ago. She kept on crying as I told her all the things in my favor—that the lump was small, and I found it early. I began to realize I had never told her about Grandma. As I explained, her question was, "Am I going to get cancer?" I had to answer. "It's a possibility, but if it happens, it will not be for years. By then, medicine may be to the point where doctors can detect it in your genes and prevent it." I continued that, on her dad's side, there is no breast cancer; perhaps her genes take after him and she will never have cancer. Deep inside, this brought up my own fears that I had had through the years. I asked her if she wanted to talk to Grandma, and she nodded. She only listened on the phone. Veronica's the kind of person who internalizes things, sets her jaw, and keeps going.

As I went through each step, talking to the surgeon, setting the surgery date, and having the surgery, I discussed each step honestly with Veronica. I'm lucky the mass was small, low-grade, and the nodes clean. I found that the better I handled things, the better Veronica could cope. The only trouble we had was that nine months prior, I had had a spinal fusion with a very difficult recovery. I was unprepared as to how long it would take me to improve; therefore, what I told Veronica did not happen. As we went through the breast cancer, Veronica's big question was, "Why do you think this is right, Mom, because look how the last surgery went?" This time, I spoke of all the possibilities, positive lymph nodes, possible chemotherapy, and hair loss. After my lumpectomy, I even took Veronica to a session of radiation.

I really felt Veronica was okay with all that happened even though she never spoke about it. However, five months later, she was at a sleepover and my phone rang. She was crying and saying, "You're okay, Mom, right? You're not going to die, right?" I reassured and calmed her. Apparently, Veronica and her friend (whose mom was carrying a high-risk pregnancy) were talking about their moms, and how they could die.

I'm glad she felt she could call. She needed reassurance and all her questions surfaced. It's so easy to tell your husband and friends that your repeat mammogram was negative and forget to tell your children.

It was recently brought to my attention that if I could sense my mother's fear, Veronica can sense my fears about back and leg pain. When I asked her, she said, "Yes, Mom, I'm scared."

My problems are small compared to those of others who may read this. Women stick together when it comes to breast cancer. Between 25 and 30 women contacted me and told me they were or knew survivors. Each call gave me additional strength, which helped me in my conversations with Veronica.

20
Robin's Hope

by Robin Martinez

How often we think it's the worst, and God means it for the best!

I know that happened to us. My husband's cancer brought him up short and turned him back to God. I'd been praying for Lusindo to be able to share my spiritual joy. He was raised Christian, and I wasn't. He had lost his faith years before and found it again in a big way; we saw so many miracles.

In November 1988, the doctor came into the hospital room with tears in his eyes and told Luch he wouldn't live to see much, if any, of 1989. Luch's adult son, Ed, was there. Ed took me aside at the elevator to tell me what the doctor had said. He was deeply upset, and I was strangely calm. "If that's what the doctor says, then we need a miracle, Ed. That's all there is to it."

I didn't think our 5-year-old son Roberto was paying attention. But as we walked back to the room, Roberto asked me, "Mom, is Dad going to die?" I got a very clear thought: "It is very important how you answer him." I took a breath and said, "Son, the doctor says Daddy will die unless God gives us a miracle."

Roberto dropped to his knees right then and there in the hallway. Now that was an odd thing; I had never told him to kneel to pray, and I don't think he had ever seen it. (We weren't churchgoers at that time, since Luch was uninterested.)

Roberto asked God very directly for a miracle and stood up. He was confident we had received it.

Later, Luch grinned at me when I sat beside him, saying, "I don't know about you, but I'm going to beat the IRS!" We both burst out laughing. How good to laugh at a time like that!

Next, Luch told me when the doctor gave him the news, his only thought was to wish he could have again the faith of his childhood. He hadn't asked for more physical life—only for God's presence in whatever life remained.

Luch lived almost 10 years from that point. So many wonderful things happened during that time. Most of all, it was enough time. Not as much as we had hoped for, but enough.

When his dad died, Roberto was 15, a young man instead of a little child. He's home-schooled, so the three of us were inseparable. (My mom called us the three musketeers.) We traveled, we camped, we enjoyed life. Our faith saw us through.

We had many adventures, medical and otherwise. How fortunate we were! Luch's cancerous kidney turned out to be operable after all—after everyone in the hospital agreed it was clearly in the liver and hopeless. I fasted for the first time in my life. It just occurred to me to do so. On the fourth day, the MRI showed the cancer was not in the liver, despite all previous evidence.

Beyond that, the only treatment Luch had was surgery for a brain metastasis and, very near the end, four months of a clinical trial at M.D. Anderson in Houston. It seemed to be turning things around. Then, suddenly, his cancer progressed again. We returned home, visited with all the family, and began to seek other treatment. Six weeks later, Lusindo died.

He was really "sick" only the last 19 days of his life. He was comatose or semi-comatose most of this time. We spent the last 12 days in hospice—a wonderful place to be after the initial shock. Thanks to hospice, Luch's pain was kept at bay. He roused to talk with family and friends.

There was always someone at his bedside; what an outpouring of love! I was with him around the clock, a great privilege. Roberto spent the last nine days at hospice, too. It was nearly an hour's trip each way from our home, and things were so touch-and-go that we didn't want to leave. Luch couldn't call for help if he needed it.

Our ever-present family was able to watch over the fellow in the next bed, too. His body began to wander in response to his wandering mind. We helped reach things for him and called the nurses for him. Once I caught him when he was falling. At first I didn't care for having a roommate. He was a blessing, though. I realized how much worse it would be to see Luch's mind go first, his body still clinging to life. Hospice was a wonderful experience for our whole family.

But it wasn't all roses. In fact, a couple of years before he died, when everything seemed medically stable, I was about to leave. I wasn't happy. However, we worked it out. Luch showed me that my presence did matter to him. (I didn't realize it, but his brain and personality were starting to deteriorate as an after-effect of post-surgical radiation. I wish I had known. The doctors never told us of the possibility until his final hospitalization.)

Another time, I was feeling distant and angry. It's a normal reaction, even though it's illogical to blame someone for an illness they can't help. Then I saw that if Luch had been given a choice between bearing his cancer or giving it to Roberto or me, he would have shouldered it without a second thought—to save us. That is love! That helped me let go of resentment and just love him.

The greatest gift from all of this is to be able to turn our pain to help others. Roberto has become such a mature person. People cannot believe he is just 15 when they meet him on AOL (America Online). He's a source of strength and friendship to so many, including me. He's smart and wise and funny. In him, Luch and I are joined, and Luch lives on. I'm so glad to have a son.

We never hid the facts from our son concerning his dad's illness. He knew from the beginning that his dad might die, and he trusted that wouldn't happen. Roberto felt absolute assurance in the miracle he asked for—and so, oddly, did we.

We were very open about the situation with our son, although no one—doctor or patient—could predict any outcome. Kidney cancer is a very individual disease with no predictable path.

As we returned for checkups and follow-up visits for Luch, Roberto even accompanied us in to see the doctor. At first it was because I wanted to be there with Luch, and we hated to leave Roberto alone in the waiting room. Roberto wanted to be with us no matter where we went. For a long while, this system worked well for us.

When Luch's cancer recurred, none of us realized exactly how serious the situation might be. That may have been fortunate. Positive attitude is one of the best weapons against recurrent cancer.

Roberto was with us when we got the news that "something" was visible in Luch's lungs. There were many tiny spots. No one could be sure from the tests that it was cancer returning. We were referred at that point to an oncologist who advised "watchful waiting."

Roberto says now that it didn't scare him. The spots were small and not frightening, and they did not change for a long time.

Later, though, Roberto began to show signs of stress from the situation. At the advice of a counselor, we began to leave him in the waiting room. Roberto didn't want to "face the music" quite so directly, yet he also felt a real fear of being kept unaware of developments. We promised we'd never lie to him, and we seemed to meet both needs. We worked to keep communications open with him, about the illness and every subject. As a result, our relationship continues to be very open to this day. I'm glad of that.

Long before Lusindo died, I joined the Internet mailing list for kidney cancer and became co-owner within a few months. It's a huge gift to me to be able to continue this work. Even though Luch is gone, his life continues to matter in a very real way to the world. Our experience (and the extensive medical education I am still receiving from it) is shared with more than 400 current members and many others who've come and gone. The work brings me healing. I hope to stay.

I wish "enough time" to all who read this. May your pain turn to good, fulfilling life work. May you and your children be blessed in unexpected ways. May your tears be turned into dancing! Despite the shadow of death, the dance of life goes on and on. Love is worth it all.

21
Amy's Year
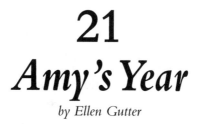
by Ellen Gutter

It's Columbus Day weekend in New England and I'm driving through the countryside with my family, taking in the lush colors of fall foliage as we travel by car down windy country roads. The car's sunroof is open as we breathe in the crisp autumn air. I'm enjoying every leaf on every tree, basking in the fullness of the season, happy to be alive.

It was just a year ago when we awaited the dreadful biopsy results. Then, we sat restlessly in Dr. David Sugarbaker's office at the Brigham and Women's Hospital in Boston to learn the diagnosis.

I was a 49-year-old Caucasian female without a history of smoking when I was diagnosed with adenocarcinoma of the lung lining. The doctors could not determine the primary site, because the cancer appeared as random cells in the right lung lining, so I was diagnosed as having ACUP (adenocarcinoma with unknown primary) at Stage 3B. Dr. Sugarbaker and his expert team at the Dana Farber Center determined the course of treatment: three rounds of chemotherapy followed by surgery resulting in the removal of the right lung, the lung lining, the diaphragm and a rib, followed by 26 rounds of radiation to the right lung cavity.

This was not looking to be a cakewalk.

My husband, Larry, immediately used the Internet to become an expert on the disease and treatment. Although a layman, he grasped all the technicalities and earned the respect of medical professionals we met while remaining a loving advocate for his wife of 13 years.

I began my journey stoically, explaining to myself that it was my job to come out the other side of this well and healed. We have an 8-year-old daughter, Amy, and I was not going to leave her motherless at this fragile age.

My family immediately pulled together and mobilized as a team. We were very open and honest with Amy about the seriousness of this illness. She felt free to ask her daddy lots of questions when he put her to bed every night. The childcaring for Amy became Larry's raison d'être as he sorted out his own feelings of sadness and anxiety. Larry maintained a full-time job with Compaq while keeping his fatherly role a top priority.

Meanwhile, my youthful parents, 72 and 77, were among my daughter's top playmates. She enjoyed their love and attention throughout the course of my recovery. Although filled with anxiety that they hid from me, they accompanied me through the medical maze to get treatments. My mother sat vigil with me during my chemo treatments, while Grandpa stayed at my house and took responsibility for getting Amy to and from her daily activities. We strove to keep Amy's life as normal as possible.

Amy's first-grade teacher, Mary Johnson, learned of my illness and immediately mobilized the school system in Amy's favor. She referred Amy to the school's psychologist, Mary Ann Burritt, whom Amy met weekly throughout the school year. For both of those women I hold a special place in my heart. They not only looked after and nurtured Amy, they gave me lots of attention, love, hope, gifts, and cards.

Among others I sought out for consoling and coaching was

my women's group of 13 years. One dear friend, Ruth Natanson, is a breast cancer survivor and offered lots of information and resources, including the Wellness Community of Newton. We learned about their Kids Count Too program, which met monthly. It offered Amy an outlet to share her concerns with and to learn from peers who were dealing with cancer in their families. Amy looked forward to these monthly gatherings and would pass up her art class to attend Kids Count Too. Concurrently, they ran parent groups, and Larry attended them all, deriving great comfort from others who were family caregivers entering this journey into the unknown.

As a driven "Type A" personality, I focused on getting well. I incorporated alternative therapies into my daily routine along with the doctor's protocol. I added Chinese herbs, meditation and visual tapes, and yoga.

I began my chemo treatments in October of 1998 and asked my friends to take turns at my bedside. That outpouring of support was so staggering that the medical facility had to find us a bigger room for the next chemo session to ensure a place for all the visitors.

Among my women's group, Gail Trubow remained as my coach with positive conviction during the whole course of my illness and recovery. She never failed to be there for me, with a hug, encouragement, or a homemade apple pie. I still remember her face when I awoke from the biopsy to learn it was cancer. She was there at my bedside holding my hand. Cathy O'Connell, who was in mid-life, changing careers from being an engineer to a pastoral counselor, peppered our talks with spiritual awakenings that offered many lessons to learn. And our beloved rabbi, Deborah Hachen of Congregation B'nai Shalom in Westboro, made herself available at a chemo session. I thank her for sitting vigil with my family and friends during my surgery.

All of these people went out of their way to let Amy know that they shared her sadness. Amy was quite aware of the frequent phone calls from friends and relatives, frequent visits from the same, and the outpouring of cards and gifts along with home-baked goodies. Amy frequently expressed how this made our family feel stronger and loved.

I later learned that the CA-125 cancer marker that read 932 before treatment began was measured at 7 after my second chemotherapy treatment. The decision was made to move to the next course of treatment, surgery. The doctor quoted discouraging statistics with regard to possible recovery. I was still determined and feeling very optimistic. The surgery was performed on February 17, 1999. A stream of family and friends stood at my bedside when I woke up in the intensive care unit. I truly believe the outpouring of love and attention that I had been receiving was life-sustaining for me. It was the greatest drug.

My mother stayed with me in intensive care night after night, attending to my wakefulness, discomfort, and overall restlessness, scratching my back where the incision had been made across my entire side, holding my hand, administering drugs, and coaxing me to eat, as food remained very unappealing to swallow. She played tag-team with my father who came during the days, and my husband who came after work until my mother arrived. I had around-the-clock family nursing. Meanwhile, my sister-in-law flew from New York City to stay at our house to take care of Amy during my hospitalization. Amy told me later that she "went easy on Aunt Lynn because she had no children of her own," and Amy did not want to make it hard for her.

I left the hospital eight days later to a house filled with flowers and cards from around the globe. Friends called religiously, then the mitzvah meals began. Donna Davis, a friend and volunteer with the Temple's Sisterhood, organized the membership to bring homemade meals every other night to our house. This went on from February through mid-August. We had moved to the neighborhood only a half-year prior to the diagnosis, and Donna called upon the neighbors as well. They, too, came with hands outstretched. My parents moved into our house for six weeks following my surgery. My husband got displaced in our bedroom by a hospital bed that my mother slept in, while I preferred the neo-natal curl on the waterbed.

My boss, a highly acclaimed CEO of research and consultancy in the computer industry, reassured me that there would be a job waiting for me, and not to compromise my health before I was ready to return.

I am weaving these vignettes about the people who were tenacious in helping me fight this sinister disease. Without them, I would have never felt the courage to move ahead. They remained my inspiration, though they'll say I was theirs. However it worked, I am filled with gratitude.

I finished radiation in August and it took until mid-September to feel myself again. I'm convinced my family came closer together and supported me at all costs, that my friends were true and ever-present for me.

Amy experienced true kinship of friendship and family throughout my illness and recovery. She learned very early to respect time, giving Mommy time to heal. She would get up early in the morning and be quiet so Mommy could sleep and heal. She also got lots of Daddy's attention to get her out on time for school or camp. Our next-door neighbor, Diane Hu, drove Amy to school all last year, acting as a surrogate mother and giving her maternal comforts.

So, as I breathe in the fresh autumn air this Columbus Day 1999, I look forward to the years ahead with a new outlook on the importance of family and friends, without whom I wouldn't have taken my next breath.

I've joined a gym and work out religiously, take long walks, and spend quality time with those I love. I've joined a weekly cancer support group at the Wellness Center and plan to return to work in a few short months. My husband just bought me new parabolic alpine skis to encourage me to meet my goal of downhill skiing this winter.

Amy remains the center of our life. Having gone through this tough year has made her more self-aware, empathetic, and confident. She expresses her feelings very easily and is not afraid to let us know when she is upset and about what.

She wrote a letter to my surgeon, Dr. Sugarbaker:

Dear Dr. Sugarbaker,

Thank you very, very, very, very, very, very, very much for saving my mother's life.

Love,

Amy Guttner

P.S. Ellen's recovery is going very well.

22

"Manuel, You Have Cancer"

by Manuel Vasquez

There is nothing more shocking than having a doctor look you in the eye and say, "You have cancer."

Back in 1994, I thought of myself as a healthy, vigorous, 55-year-old man. I had plenty of energy, and I felt just great! Then, Bingo!

I had gone in for a long overdue medical checkup at my wife's insistence, although my overall health was good. Suddenly, we had to take action on two problems. One was a pre-cancerous condition involving polyps in the colon; the other was a life-threatening localized prostate cancer.

So there I was, in total disbelief, feeling perfectly fine, with no symptoms whatsoever, wondering what to do next. The Human Resources Department of the company I worked for referred me to someone who had already dealt with the same kind of cancer. I left a message on his voicemail, wondering if my call would be returned. Within a few hours, I received a response saying: "Manuel, hi buddy! This is Bob Moore...I am calling you from Brazil!" He spoke to me as a survivor, not as a professional making a diagnosis. He knew exactly what to say to shake me out of my perplexity and empower me to explore with my doctor the best treatment decision for me.

The after-effects of prostate cancer treatment may affect

the essence of how you perceive yourself as a man, your quality of life, your marriage, and your family. I recovered from the
treatment just fine. However, I found myself supremely frustrated, depressed, and *very, very angry!* My life was saved
just in time, but its quality, as a result of sexual impotency,
had left a vacuum. Because of my feelings of overwhelming
anger, I withdrew affection from my wife, and I began estrang-
ing myself emotionally from her, due to my perceived incapac-
ity to express physical intimacy. You can imagine the effect of
this depression in my professional life as well.

In the process of sorting out my thoughts and feelings, I
remembered my newly found comrade, Bob Moore, reaching
out to me from his remote assignment. If a total faceless
stranger were able to reach out from several thousand miles
away and affect my life, why couldn't I do the same, right here
in my own community?

The opportunity arose from the American Cancer Society
Patient Services program. In it, I discovered there are nearly
200,000 men every year who, in the face of prostate cancer
diagnosis, need information, the exchange of experiences, a
safe buddy for emotional release, and empowerment to
choose with his physician the correct treatment decision to
take charge of their lives.

The American Cancer Society Man to Man program, in
which I am involved, is an organized way of reaching out to
men with prostate cancer. If these services were not organized, many people would not be reached.

I receive much more out of my involvement than I put into
it. As a result, and to my surprise, I found that reaching out
to others got me out of my self-destructive, overwhelming
anger. In the process of releasing that negative force, my abil-

ity to give physical and emotional affection was restored. In hindsight, the metamorphosis would not have occurred had I not been involved in reaching out to others.

Another step on my road to emotional recovery was to be able to communicate my apprehensions, fears, and emotions to my own offspring. Fortunately, all of my six children were adults at the time of my diagnosis and treatment. That makes a big difference. It is a lot easier to communicate with adult children, and to tell-it-like-it-is, than to have to "dress it up" for the small fry. I was spared the agony of having to deal with little ones. As a matter of fact, it was very comforting to be able to discuss openly, and as adults, the life-changing, and potentially lethal events, that were about to take place. Their support was a source of strength for which I am deeply grateful.

To complete the cycle, I had to discuss with my male children the genetic implications of the dreaded disease. Intergenerational transmission of certain cancers appears to be a reality, and it must be dealt with. Not a pleasant task, but an essential one for which they must prepare themselves. By taking responsibility for their own lives through behavior modification (diet, exercise, early detection, etc.), that may indeed reduce their probabilities of contracting the disease. Science appears to be at the threshold of making transcendental discoveries in the area of genetics. Until that time finally comes, we must be on the lookout.

23

Children's Support Group Was a Godsend

by Angela and Barry Wilkerson

Angela:

I'm a mom, and I stay at home with my daughter, Kassie, 15; and sons, Justin, 13, and Tommy, 6.

I found out right after Tommy was born that I had melanoma. It was superficial, so I had it removed. The following year, I had more biopsies because my lymph nodes had started to swell. The doctors told me I had lymphoma leukemia. So, I thought: Okay, we'll do the chemo, and I'll get on with my life. They said, "No, we can't do that. You have a slow-growing cancer that can't be cured. We can treat it, but we can't cure you. We're going to put you on 'watch and wait.'" That means watch me, and when I get sick enough, start the treatment.

When we told our children, five years ago, they were so young. I had lost my mom to cancer when I was 16, so I wanted to be up front with my kids. And I don't know if that was the best thing to do because they didn't understand. Now, finally, they're saying, "Well, what's this all about? What do you have? You have lymphoma. What's that?"

Kassie understands now, but Justin is still confused about what I have and what it means. We told them that there's no cure now, but we hope that within my lifetime, they'll find a cure. So it's just an everyday thing for them. They've been living with this for five years, and I was sick on and off for a long time. It was just normal for them to see me on the couch sleeping. I did go out of the country for nine weeks. I'll let Barry, my husband, tell you how that was, being alone with the kids.

Barry:

Angela went out of the country over the Christmas holidays for some experimental treatment. The children held up very well. Tommy, the youngest one, didn't really know why she was gone, but the older two, although missing her, viewed this for the best and took it pretty well. It was a time that was spent in reflection and for bonding among the three kids and me. I guess they've just now become aware of the fact that potentially it's a fatal disease. And our middle son, Justin, is just now starting to raise some questions like, "What kind of cancer is it?" although we've told him many times.

His friend next door, Brad, has Hodgkins disease. You can just see Justin's curiosity in asking him questions about it because of the similarity between Brad's disease and his mom's disease. He's making jokes about jumping on the trampoline and having his hair fall out! He's just now starting to ask some pretty grown-up questions about the disease and some of the treatments.

Angela:

It could be that Barry and I just went too fast, and Justin couldn't handle it. But now he's able to acknowledge what's going on. I remember him lying in bed when he was little, crying, "I don't want you to die." Now, he doesn't know if we were too honest with him at the time. I do believe in being honest with my kids, because my parents weren't honest with us about my mom. It was devastating to us.

Some days are really great, and there's a lot of energy. And some days... There was a period of time when I was really sick. Luckily, Barry's work was so slow that he took over my job and didn't go to work.

And now I'm starting traditional treatment, so the kids are seeing a different part of this cancer. They're seeing me lose my hair a little bit. Previously, I'd always sought out alternative medicine. So I've always been going to practitioners and taking lots of pills. The kids just accept that Mom's weird—she takes all these pills and she eats strange food. We've learned to like whole-wheat breads, organic foods, and some things that the kids still haven't developed a taste for, but those foods have become part of our menu, so the kids are somewhat adjusted to it.

When I learned of the support group for kids at Porter Adventist Hospital, I thought it was a godsend. This is something I would have loved to have had as a kid myself. I immediately put my kids in the group because of what had happened when I was a child. It still affects me. (I was 11 when my mom was first diagnosed and 16 when she died.) To date, the kids have been in the support group for four years. They look forward to it so much that they have forgone a lot of other activities.

It's so important to be honest with your children, to give them the information they want. Kids have vivid imaginations. If you don't give them some sort of direction, they'll just go all over the place. I think that's worse than anything else.

A lot of people think their kids are tough. I've suggested to other people that they put their kids in a support group. They say, "Oh, no. They're fine. They're handling it." But they may be ignoring their kids. They may have no idea what their kids are going through. And I think it takes someone who has been through it to know what kids are going to go through. You can't ignore it, and you have to include them along the way, such as in trying on your wigs. That's what we just did last week. I ordered a box of wigs, and my boys were putting the wigs on. Tommy even put them on the dog! It was great fun.

The support group for the kids made all the difference. It truly has been a godsend.

24

There Is a Purpose to All This

by Juli Brennan

When I discovered I had breast cancer, the impact on my family was overwhelming! When I returned from the doctor's office, I sat down with my three kids, Sara, 13; Megan, 10; and Matt, 8, and talked with them about my illness.

My wonderful husband, Tom, was there all the way. He was able to take a lot of vacation time, which took a big load off our shoulders. When I was in the hospital or had doctor's appointments, the kids had questions, and they tended to ask him more than they would ask me, because I would just cry. As a family, we were really honest with them. Young Matt had a really hard time getting it all. We tried to keep the conversation age-appropriate. The girls had seen my aunt as a 35-year breast cancer survivor, and their grandpa has prostate cancer. So they knew some of the terminology and some of what was going on, but it sure brought out a lot of questions. We cried and prayed a lot.

We just survived my first year with breast cancer. I did five months of chemotherapy. I had a recurrence in December and went back and forth with tests, MRIs, and what-not, and ended up having a mastectomy.

I was a speech-and-hearing assistant for three and a half years. In January, I decided it was time that I stayed home. I always worked part time and with children. My kids have grown up with my working part time, but we're sure all glad not to be so scheduled now.

Throughout it all, what was very helpful to the children and me was keeping a routine. They had lots of questions! We always answered them honestly. Any changes, and they were informed. It was also fun to be a family and to go do family fun! We all kept a great sense of humor throughout this ordeal.

A friend told us about a kids' support group. I was very hesitant at first and thought, "Is this going to be worse? Is this going to frighten them?" I was a Stage Two. I knew that some parents there were sicker than I was. So I had those reservations. After I was reassured, then the kids had reservations. They weren't really sure what a support group was all about. Afterward, it ended up being the best thing we ever did for them. Besides the activities, there was proper supervision and a lot of care and compassion for them. The staff knew what was appropriate and how much they could take. My kids made some good friends. And even if they didn't talk about cancer per se, being with other kids, if they wanted to talk about it, was great, and if they didn't, that was okay.

I think taking the kids with me to a couple of doctor's appointments also helped. And after the surgery, they came into my room. The doctor happened to be in there too, and it was very reassuring because he was very open and honest with them, as were we.

It has been a very tough year, but I was amazed at my kids and their strength, courage, and faith. It was overwhelming. We got through it, and we're going to keep chugging along.

We continued to go to church. Our family and friends were

there for us. The whole experience brought us back to "what's really important."

I was fortunate in another way. The teachers at my kids' school were wonderful. In the middle of summer, they'd come over and take my kids for the day when I had chemo. They'd take them to the movies, or they made meals for me. It was so nice.

I weathered my treatment (surgery) better than most, and with the remission, I feel blessed. I am always humbled by the outpouring of care, concern, and prayers I received.

Mostly, I'm thankful for my family and each day I have with them. Our Lord does answer prayers—and I learned the power of prayer!

I know there is a purpose to all this experience.

Laugh, love, live!

25

Teachers Can Make a Big Difference

by Kathy Anthony

When I was diagnosed with breast cancer, it was absolutely devastating for my family. I think shock is the best way to describe it. My mother had breast cancer, as did her three sisters, so I wasn't shocked. Everyone else was. It was a surprise, but it's not so unexpected. I just said, "Okay, well, let's do what we need to do and get on with life." When I was informed of my diagnosis my husband was out of town and wouldn't be back until the next day. That was really pretty devastating in and of itself. At the time, my daughter, Kelsey, was in fourth grade. She had just turned 10, and I was going to lose a breast just as she was getting them. That made it very difficult. All the hormones were starting to run in her, and you never know how to approach kids.

Because I didn't know if I was going to come apart at the seams or not, a good friend who had come with me to the doctor's office suggested she spend the night at my house. Meanwhile, I had to decide how to tell my daughter, but I decided I needed a little bit of breathing space. My daughter knew I didn't feel well, had been at the doctor's office, but didn't know what to make of it. I felt I needed to come to grips with it.

I had taught high-school math and science for 10 years. I quit teaching when we adopted Kelsey as an infant, so I haven't been in the teaching game for that long. I still volunteer in the schools, so another friend who was a teacher at Kelsey's school said, "There's a skate night at school. I'm a chaperone; I'll take her." And not only did she take her to the skate night, she kept her overnight!

I spent the night getting myself together. The next day I went to school and told my daughter's teacher about the diagnosis and that I needed to talk to Kelsey. The principal graciously gave us a conference room. I wanted Kelsey to know what was going on because I had another doctor's appointment that day. My teacher friend was taking her again that night, and she had a right to know what the situation was. Kelsey is adopted; we've always been up front with her about the adoption, and I felt I needed to be up front with her about this. It wasn't as if she were 6 or 7 years old and couldn't get it. Mom's a science teacher and science-oriented. Kelsey is science-oriented and she was capable of understanding this. She knew another little girls whose mother had been diagnosed with breast cancer two years earlier. Thus, she was aware, to a certain extent, of what it involved: that Mom would be really sick and very tired.

We sat down in the conference room, and I sat her on my lap, and I told her. I reminded her that her grandmother had had breast cancer and had died 20 years after that diagnosis of something else; that her great aunt lived 25 years after her diagnosis and died of something else. And two other great aunts were still alive and had kicked the breast cancer (their worst problems were things like arthritis and stomach pains). And I said, "You know what? Mom's gonna go through the same things, except with the benefit of modern medicine. And I'm gonna die in 40 years of something else. And we're gonna fight it, and we're gonna win this battle!"

At first, I think, she wasn't sure that what she was hearing was reality. She cried a little bit. Then she said, "What do we have to do?" I told her right then what she could do the most for me was to be supportive. If I needed to go to the doctor, and I needed to leave her with somebody to get her homework done, then she should cooperate with that person while I was away. Then she would meet and talk with my surgeon and my other doctors, and we would go from there. When I knew more details, I would tell her and I would answer her questions. To me, that was really important. She didn't know what questions to ask, initially, but I had to give her the chance to ask them.

When I finished talking with her, I told her that she didn't have to go back to class right away, that I had told her teacher that I was very sick, and that her teacher understood it might take a while before Kelsey went back to the classroom. She asked me to come back to her class with her for a little bit, which I did.

One thing that helped was that Kelsey knew another student in her class whose mother was going through treatment for cancer. The teacher already had one student going through this. So Kelsey said, "Well, Alex and I might have to stick together." I don't think they really talked a lot during that school year, but it gave them a little bit of a bond just to know that each other's mom had cancer and was going through chemotherapy and radiation. As the teacher told me later, "They're wearing their emotions on their sleeves. They cry if someone looks at them cross-eyed. But they're going to be okay."

The one thing that I feel really strongly about is that school districts should prepare teachers to deal with kids whose parents have catastrophic illnesses. This teacher was phenomenal. She had two grown kids, one who had been very sick as a child—not with cancer though. But nothing had prepared her, or any other teacher in that school, for kids who walk into their classroom and cry in the middle of a math lesson because they're thinking Mom might die on the operating table. That's an area we need to tackle: to get some kind of training for teachers with students in these circumstances.

Then, another mom who has cancer told me about a support group for children at a local hospital. That convinced me that this was a place that I wanted to put my daughter. I had to fight with my husband, who resists anything that smacks of "shrink." I said, "Well, if we're going to make a mistake, I'd rather make this kind of mistake than not do anything." After Kelsey's year in the group, he concluded, "That was the best thing we ever did for her." It really made a difference in her ability to deal with it.

We introduced her to the surgeon and the oncologist, and she came to one meeting with each of them. She missed school the day I had surgery for a modified radical mastectomy (which was followed by 30 weeks of chemotherapy, followed by six weeks of radiation). She stayed in the waiting room with her dad. I had given her a stuffed animal before my surgery. I think that helped. The Beanie Babies were really becoming the fad, so I gave her the kangaroo with the baby in the pouch. I told her, just as the mom took care of that baby, I was going to take care of her, and I'd see her after surgery.

The first thing she asked my surgeon when he walked out was, "Did you sing my mother to sleep?" We had heard that he was in a barber shop quartet of doctors, and I had asked him the same thing as they wheeled me into the operating room, "Are you going to sing me to sleep?" He said, "No, there's a new team in here. I'm training them today. I can't."

But it was a clear indication of how Kelsey was handling it.

Also, I really appreciated the nurses in the chemotherapy unit in my oncologist's office. Kelsey had come to chemotherapy one time, and she was really hesitant about that. She hates needles. To sit in a room with all these people undergoing chemotherapy was like death. When she got there, the nurses asked her if she wanted a cookie and some pop. She asked them a lot of questions, and they answered all of them. When she saw that I wasn't going to look like death warmed over in there, and that after chemotherapy I'd be okay for several hours, she felt reassured. It was the next day that I was really sick. She understood that when I went there, I wasn't in pain all the time; neither was everyone else. Some patients were pretty sick, but it wasn't a foreign place any more. It wasn't just some place she'd heard about. She actually saw it. I think that was important to her.

The radiation therapist did the same thing, and that really helped. She got to see the machine that tattooed me. They even showed her how they make the blocks to block out the radiation.

Because my daughter is really artsy, I decided to involve her in getting hats and things like that. I told her that I needed my fashion consultant to come with me. It was before my hair fell out. We went hat shopping for an afternoon, and that generated a lot of questions in a non-threatening way. It was really good for us. She also came along when I picked out a wig. My husband came, too. The sales lady let her try on other wigs. She tried hairpieces, hats, and turbans. You name it, she tried it. I think that really helped her to accept Mom as bald, Mom with a wig, Mom with a turban. That really is the crux of it for a lot of kids. They don't want their friends to see their parents bald, especially if it's their mother. In private though, my daughter wanted to rub my head.

Throughout the ongoing ordeal, the key has been honesty. I've taught kids long enough in junior high and high school to know Kelsey was old enough. I felt I needed to answer her questions, not bombard her with too many details that she couldn't understand and that would just cause her to worry. Providing age-appropriate answers was important.

Now, a year later, Kelsey is helping other kids in the support group. It clearly shows how essential that activity is to helping kids cope.

26
Andy Updates
by Susan Stadnik

Author's Note: *After Susan Stadnik's husband, Andy, was diagnosed with cancer, each evening for 128 days she e-mailed "Andy Updates" to "literally hundreds of friends and co-workers." The following provides excerpts of this thoughtful journal, mostly as it relates to their three children, now 8, 6, and 4.*

5/1/98

I am very sad to report that Andy was diagnosed last night with acute myeloid leukemia, M-5. The day before, we were told that it was not leukemia; however, after highly specialized tests at NIH, the diagnosis was confirmed. We are transferring by ambulance today to the Acute Leukemia Center at Georgetown to begin chemotherapy.

5/6/98

The highlight of the day was a visit from the kids. Unfortunately for Sam (Samantha), she could not go on the ward (you must go through an airlock) because chicken pox are going around her class. She was crushed. Sam stayed with Grandma and Grandpa Lee in the lobby while Alex (Alexandria) and Matt visited Daddy. It was a little scary entering through the airlock, scrubbing their hands, and then putting on a mask. They were happy to see Daddy, but you could see they were very worried and concerned.

They brought a wonderful banner that Alex and her classmates made in art class, plus many other cards and drawings. They kept the masks (we gave one to Sam!), and they were excited about taking them home to play doctor.

5/9/98

We hooked up the videophones, and Andy and I have made several calls home where my parents are taking care of the kids. The kids love it! The picture quality isn't the greatest, but it is so good for Alex, Matt, and Sam to see and hear Daddy.

5/10/98

I was able to go home for a few hours for a Mother's Day dinner with the kids and my parents. It was great to be home, but I felt a little out of place; "home" has become room B2007 at Georgetown. My mom and dad are doing an amazing job with Alex, Matt, and Sam; no one knows better than I what a tough job that is.

5/13/98

Ironically, I have been a registered bone marrow donor for five years. I registered because I felt I should offer to help others in case someone in my family ever needed help. I get chills thinking of the day I went to have blood taken to be typed for the registry. I took Alex and Matt with me (Matt was a baby), and talked to Alex about what I was doing and told her that I also donate blood regularly. It was one of life's little lessons that has turned out to mean so much. It really means a lot now for Alex, Matt, and Sam to know that other people are giving blood, platelets, and potentially bone marrow to help their daddy get better.

5/14/98

I picked up Sam from school today—the first time since Andy has been in the hospital. She was thrilled to have a special afternoon with Mommy. We ate ice cream cones, then skipped all the way to the toy store where she picked out a special toy. She also picked out something for Alex and Matt, plus a surprise for Daddy... a pop-up eyeball. (The doctors love it!)

5/15/98

The Consumer Product Safety Commission did its part to improve public safety by descending on Georgetown and cheering Andy on to a speedy recovery. Approximately 40 wonderful co-workers showed up with banners and balloons outside of Andy's window this afternoon. It was an amazing show of support and meant a lot to Andy. He works with an incredible group of people who have demonstrated they will do just about anything to let him know they care.

5/23/98

I am writing this Andy update from the Stadnik's Family Georgetown Slumber Party! Alex, Matt, Sam, and I are staying in the Leavey Conference Center right here on campus in the building next to Andy's. Grandma and Grandpa Lee dropped off the kids so we could have our evening together. Alex, Matt, and Sam waved to Daddy outside his window; Alex performed cartwheels and back walkovers, much to Andy's delight. He gave a "thumbs up" and a wave goodbye, and we went next door to have our slumber party. It was the first time in four weeks that I have spent a night with the kids. Andy is spending the night alone but is happy the four of us are in the next building.

5/24/98

The Stadnik Family Georgetown Slumber Party was a great success! The kids and I enjoyed a fun evening together in the hotel next to Andy's building. It was so good for the kids to ask me questions and talk more about what is happening to Daddy. Before they left, we stopped by the airlock on Andy's floor. He met us at the door and gave them all high-fives through the glass. Andy was fine without me, but he is happy to have me back in the room for the remainder of this first round of treatment.

6/2/98

On the day Andy was released from the hospital, I picked up Alex and Matt, and my parents picked up Sam from ballet. I went to the hospital to get Andy while everyone hurried to put up banners and balloons! (Balloons and banners, kindness of our friends at Bethesda Country Day School!) Around 6 p.m. we came honking into the cul-de-sac, and the neighborhood went wild. I still can't believe it.

This was a big day for Andy, and indeed for the entire family. We know he has a lot ahead of him, and he knows we need to take things one day at a time. We have an emergency bag by the door just in case we need to go to the hospital in a hurry (just like when I was pregnant!). Grandma and Grandpa Lee are staying, so we have lots of hands to help. I don't know what we would have done without them these past five weeks. They have been amazing and have stepped in and completely taken over running the house. They didn't miss a beat! Many of you have seen them in the carpool line, at soccer games, at gymnastics practice, or at the swimming pool. The kids are crazy about them, and I think they are a big reason that Alex, Matt, and Sam have been able to handle the situation so well. Mom and Dad, you're the best!!

6/21/98

Back in the hospital, Andy had a Father's Day visit from Alex, Matt, and Sam today. They brought Daddy homemade cards and were excited to see him. They thought his Hickman input line was cool and were glad to see that it was no longer in his neck. We had planned on having lunch in the room with Andy, but with the severity of his nausea, lunch is the last thing on his mind. So the kids, my mom, and I had lunch in the cafeteria before they headed back home. Although this is still very hard for the kids, knowing that Daddy will come home soon is a big comfort.

8/1/98

Back at home, Andy and I celebrated our anniversary today. Eleven years! We spent the afternoon at the pool with the kids. While we were in the water, Andy sat by the pool enjoying the nice weather and watching the kids have fun.

8/4/98

Andy is back in the hospital for surgery.

8/26/98

This afternoon we got the call that Andy could come home again! I headed back to Georgetown. Packing up the room was no small task, considering we made ourselves right at home by bringing the laptop, printer, and other necessities. The ice cream, of course, came with us, and is one of the few things Andy can eat.

Just because we are home does not mean that Andy is back to his old self again. That will take some time. We had been home all of five minutes when he started throwing up. But what better place to be sick than in the comfort of your own home?! The kids are great and brought Daddy water and his medicine. I heard Matt ask my dad tonight as he was getting ready for bed, "Grandpa, is Daddy staying home tonight or does he have to go back to the hospital?" When my dad said he was staying home, Matt asked with excitement, "You mean forever?!!" He jumped for joy and ran to tell his sisters. In their own way, they know Daddy is better but that he could get sick again. For now, he is home; all three of the kids are sleeping better tonight. What an ordeal this has been for them. I don't know what we would have done without my mom and dad to provide stability and love at home for the past four months while Andy and I were away.

8/30/98

Andy is feeling a little stronger and is starting to settle into a routine. For this and other reasons, I have made the difficult decision to change the Andy Updates from daily to periodically. After 122 consecutive days, it will be hard for all of us not to have the daily update.

However, I feel the time is right to change. Tomorrow I start a new job. I will be working full time at Norwood as the school's database manager. I am very excited, and it means a lot to work some place I care so much about. In addition, Sam starts school tomorrow—a big 4-year-old in the pre-kindergarten class at Bethesda Country Day School! Alex starts third grade and Matt starts first grade on September 8 at Norwood.

10/27/98

This evening was much like many evenings at the Stadnik house. Alex, Matt, and I arrived home after a late day at school and work to find Andy curled up on the couch, half sleeping, half fighting the effects of the IL-2 treatments. Sammy was reading books in a newly constructed fort across the room from Andy. Having Daddy sick on the couch has become a normal part of her life.

Andy was too sick to join us for dinner, so as with most nights the kids and I sat down at the table together. I was sitting next to Matt and gently broke the news that one of his tadpoles died. He has been raising two tadpoles since this summer and has been carefully and eagerly watching their journey from polliwog to frog. He was crushed and soon had huge tears coming out of his eyes. They seemed to be coming from the very core of his being. He climbed into my lap and cried for several minutes.

I was surprised at the strength of his emotion but sensed he was crying about more than just his tadpole. Last week, his favorite fish, Ropey, died in our aquarium. He was upset, but not like this.

Alex and Sam were concerned to see their brother so upset. Sam helpfully suggested that we could pour some water on the tadpole and he wouldn't be dead anymore. Alex and Matt immediately said no, that wasn't true, and I gently explained to Sammy that once something or someone dies, they do not come back. We talked about heaven and being with God, and that Mr. Tadpole, or someone who dies, cannot come back and be with us again.

This concerned Sam, and she helpfully suggested that our dog Yukon, who was keeping his vigil for food fallen from the dinner table, would never die. I said that yes, someday he would. Sam maintained that no, he wouldn't. "Our neighbor's dog just died, but she was very old," she said. "Yukon is new, so he won't die." Alex and Matt listened uncomfortably as I explained the unpleasant reality in a gentle way to Sam.

Sam asked about people, and when she heard that people die and don't come back, she told us that we'd all die on the same day. As I addressed this, she had reached the absorption level of a 4 1/2-year-old and started blowing bubbles in her milk.

While we were talking about this, Alex covered her ears and said she did not want to talk about it any more. She suggested we take a vote and not talk about the "D word" anymore tonight. Matt leaned over to me and whispered in my ear. "The 'D word' is 'dying.'" "Everyone who wants to stop talking about the 'D word' raise your hand!" Three hands went up immediately, and they all looked at me. I shot my hand up into the air with a big smile, wiped Matt's tadpole tears, and said let's have dessert.

After dinner, while Andy was still sick on the couch, the four of us climbed into bed and read *The Tenth Good Thing About Barney*. This was Matt's choice. It's about a little boy whose cat dies. We also read *When Eric's Mom Fought Cancer* and *The Jester Has Lost His Jingle*. As we cuddled in my bed, they paid great attention to the stories, commenting on how Eric's situation was similar to their own and how mad they are at cancer. Sam pointed out that Daddy doesn't have cancer, he has leukemia (pronouncing it better than many adults). Matt informed her that Daddy does have cancer, because leukemia means that you have cancer in your blood.

We turned out the lights, and I told them stories about when I was little (one of their favorite subjects!). I told them about my duck Barney and how sad I was when he died. We also talked about happy stories, and they drifted off to sleep.

I lay there in the dark marveling at how their childhood has changed. A normal evening in our house is so different from that of other children. I share this experience to give a better picture of how Andy's illness has changed all of us. When you see Alex laughing and running on the soccer field, you would never guess that she is scared to death that her daddy might die. Or Matt, who while mourning a tadpole is expressing his deepest fear that Daddy could die, too. The kids are adjusting well and have a tremendous amount of support, but tonight made me realize again that while they appear to be tough on the outside, they are really very fragile on the inside.

Andy is feeling very sick from the Interleukin-2 shots. He has a few hours worth of energy per day, and then he is wiped out. Lately he has felt worse, but this is all to be expected. He has huge, painful welts at the injection sites. He goes to the doctor tomorrow for a checkup and then must head back to

Georgetown on Monday for three more days of high-dose injections. All of our spirits remain high because we refuse to let this get the best of us.

1/29/99

REMISSION!!!

We just heard from Andy's doctor, and all the tests show he is in remission. Obviously, this is great news, and we are thrilled! Andy will talk to his doctor next week about starting back to work—at least part time—very soon. He also has big plans to start running again, and he is eager to get back to his pre-leukemia shape.

This is a huge hurdle, but Andy will continue to have biopsies every three months for two years. He will also see his doctor at the Lombardi Cancer Center and have blood work done once a month. We will take things one step at a time and are enjoying this long-awaited good news. The five of us are headed out for a special celebration complete with hot fudge sundaes all around! Thank you all for your continued support. It truly has been a team effort. I will continue to keep you posted and look forward to future updates filled with good news.

Go Andy!

27

Helping Kids CLIMB through Tough Times

by David Scales, Middletown Press correspondent

Marli Roblee has to wake up a little earlier than most to commute to her job at Aetna. Her first stop is the Middlesex Hospital Cancer Center in Middletown, Connecticut for radiation treatment to prevent her breast cancer from returning. After her diagnosis in 2003, she was unsure how much to tell her nine-year-old son Jeffrey, but a solution appeared when Roblee hosted a field trip and learned of a new outpatient program, Children's Lives Include Moments of Bravery (CLIMB), at the Middlesex Hospital Cancer Center.

The free, six-week program is designed to help children of parents or grandparents with cancer deal with the emotional stress the disease can cause. Parent orientation begins at the first meeting with subsequent meetings targeted toward the children. After dinner, an hour and a half of discussing a feeling they call "the emotion of the week" begins to help them understand their feelings.

"It's a learning experience for the child," Roblee said. "It's learning in the sense that it takes away the fear of the unknown. We can handle anything if we know about it."

By using art and crafts, the kids learn how to calm their anxiety about a family member's illness. One exercise is to make a paper box, which is called a "strongbox." On the box are pictures of things the children make to help them feel better, such as sports, music, friends, etc. After it's finished, they put inside little slips of paper with their worries written on them. The idea behind the box is the worry slips deposited inside and the positive pictures on the outside help children literally place their fear in a box of their own strength.

"Jeffrey put in a couple of worry slips like 'I'm afraid my mom and dad are going to die,'" Roblee said. "He had my husband and me fill out worry slips, and once you put the worry slip in the box, they're not weighing on your mind. They're not weighing on you."

Roblee discovered a lump on her breast. Thinking it was a cyst, a biopsy was done. She was diagnosed with breast cancer in December 2003, and it was confirmed as malignant in January 2004.

Roblee had many questions. "How do I tell my son? How can I keep him from being afraid? I don't want to tell him too much, but how much is enough?" Roblee said. "That's where CLIMB is fantastic!"

The program doesn't stop with art and crafts; kids are also familiarized with the equipment used to treat cancer. Jeffrey was shown the room where his mother undergoes radiation treatments and was encouraged by the new weapons in the anti-cancer arsenal.

"He's asking me questions when he has concerns and it's not just this glassy-eyed look," Roblee said. "Now he understands more and we can talk about it and I'm able to reassure him that everything's going to be fine."

When not in class at John Lyman Middle School in Middlefield, exercising his love of math, Jeffrey lends a hand at home.

"I've been helping her in the house and I've been getting things she shouldn't be getting up for," Jeffrey said. "I lift things like laundry baskets. It's tough to know that my mom had cancer and now we're getting through it and it's all better."

Roblee said because of CLIMB, the lines of communication between her and Jeffrey are open wider than before. Jeffrey has begun to teach his mother how to snowboard. He also said she does pretty well on powdery snow, but tends to wipe out on icy slopes.

Wendy Peterson is an advanced practice registered nurse, specializing in psychiatry and psycho-oncology, who runs the program. She said the goal is to help children find ways to cope with strong feelings associated with having a sick family member. Parents are also given support to help speak with their children if fears and questions arise.

"When somebody has cancer, people normally get upset," Peterson said. "It's normal for a family's life to be disrupted, it's normal for children to have feelings, and it's necessary for children to express how they feel and have age-appropriate information."

Anne Campbell-Maxwell, administrative director for the cancer center, discovered The Children's Treehouse Foundation, a nonprofit organization in Denver, Colo. Basing it on their model, CLIMB has gained some national attention. She recently returned from a national psycho-oncology meeting (APOS) where the CLIMB program was introduced to a national audience by The Children's Treehouse Foundation founder, Peter van Dernoot.

The six-week pilot program finished in December, and another is beginning, and hopes are high for a continuation. Jeffrey and Marli said they would both love to come back.

Peterson remains hopeful that the program will not only be able to continue, but expand. The group will have a reunion in April.

"We're really trying to increase awareness so that more children can be referred to the program," Peterson said. "Our ultimate goal is to increase the participation of the children and we're also developing a concurrent parent program. The parent program will be focused on giving parents information about what is age-appropriate information to give children because children have different cognitive abilities depending upon their age."

Roblee hopes to keep hitting the slopes and one day see Jeffery get his license, go to his prom, and rock her grandchildren. She is currently undergoing reconstructive surgery.

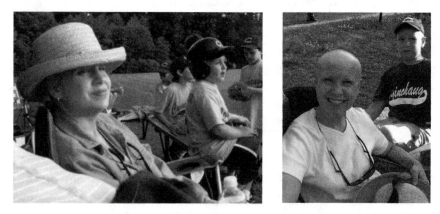

Marli Roblee during chemo treatment, with and without chapeau,
enjoying her son, Jeff, during a baseball game.

Part III

Children: Expressing Themselves

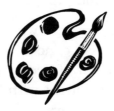

28
From Gilda's Club

by Laura Dirmish, C.S.W.

I currently run a program for children whose parents are living with cancer. In addition to the supportive work I do with the children, I find myself spending a good deal of time educating and supporting the parents of these children. I am always looking for resources the parents can take with them to refer to whenever they feel the need.

Two of my children decided they wanted to share their experiences with other children.

Anna Pelavin is a 10-year-old whose mother has been living with metastatic breast cancer since Anna was 6. Her mother is unable to get out of bed or spend much time with her daughters. Anna is eloquent with her experience, able to verbalize her thoughts and fears.

Chaya Rosner is a 9-year-old whose mother died of lymphoma in February. Chaya's mother was living with lymphoma for four years.

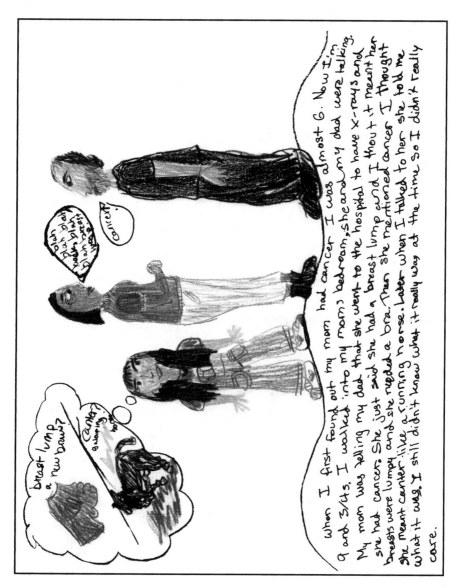

Anna Pelavin (10 years old)

She was 6 years old when her mother was diagnosed with breast cancer.

New York City

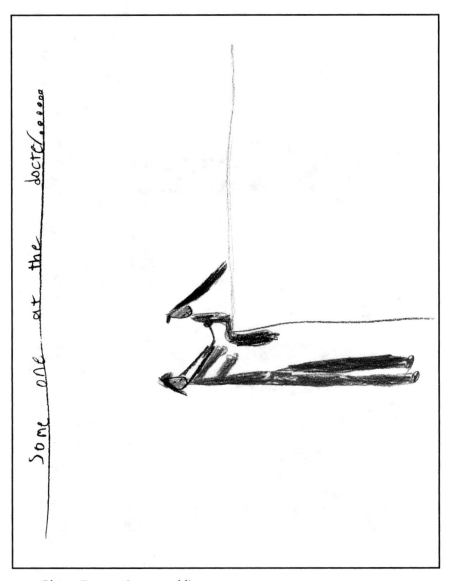

Chaya Rosner (9 years old)

She was 5 years old when her mother was diagnosed with Lympnoma.

Mom died February, 1999

New York City

29

Mom's Cancer

by Susie Klodnicki (age 11; 9 when this began)

I was seated at the kitchen table picking at the skin on the tips of my fingers. My parents wanted to tell me something. Some news. Good news? I didn't know, but I was nervous.

My muscles tightened when my dad started to speak. It was around Thanksgiving. Dad was telling my brother and me that when my mom went to the doctor, she found out something was wrong. She had been having an enormous pain in her back on the left side. The doctor took an x-ray and had found a blob the size of a softball. I did know about my mom's pain, but it was a small matter. Now I was truly worried.

A month later we found out Mom had lung cancer. She had to have a biopsy, a test to see if you have cancer by taking samples of your tissue. We got to talk to my mom a little bit, but she couldn't remember that well. She asked us three times where we had gone for lunch!

She would need surgery unless the radiation, chemotherapy, and medicine got completely rid of that awful glob (which I now know is called a tumor).

For the following month and a half, my mom had chemotherapy—which is getting pumped full of drugs to kill the cancer cells—and radiation—which is like getting zapped. Then in February, she got her lymph nodes taken out to see if the cancer had spread to any other part of her body. The results said the cancer hadn't spread.

On March 3, my mom went to the hospital. That day she was having surgery. My dad dropped us off at school and went to the hospital with my mom. That night, we had someone stay with us and my dad spent the night at the hospital. I was so scared. I knew my mom could die.

The next night someone else spent the night with us. But the next night Dad was home. I bombarded him with questions, and he answered them the best he could.

Every day we visited Mom. It was creepy seeing Mom tired and weak in the hospital bed. It was during the Winter Olympics, and I can still remember one night we stayed late. I was hungry, and we walked down the hall to the vending machines. There was a really cool one that had different flavored popcorn. I think I chose the white cheddar, but it came out jalapeño flavored.

As it got closer to the time when Mom could leave the hospital, we went on walks down the halls. My dad had a special case to put communion wafers in so he could take it to the hospital and give it to Mom. My mom looked small and not strong and had an IV in her arm. I admired her for being so brave.

Finally, on March 13, she came home from the hospital. I was as happy as a poor person finding a money tree. We still had to be very careful around Mom. Now she has started taking pain medicine and having physical therapy. Usually people with cancer lose their hair before surgery. But my mom was losing it after surgery. It was weird when she got a wig.

Earlier when the doctors were looking for the cause of Mom's cancer, they suspected smoking. My mom had smoked very little, then she found out it was bad and quit a long time ago. The doctors were not sure if it was the cause, but that just shows you how bad smoking is.

Soon Mom was not going to the doctor so often. And her hair was growing back! It had been long months since everything was normal. I gave my mom back rubs so it would ease the pain. She still can't do certain things because of her surgery, but she is doing fine with one lung and four fewer ribs.

I'm so happy she is safe and sound today.

30
Mom Talked With Me Every Day

by Mica Fulgham

I'm 14 and two years ago, my mom was diagnosed with cervical cancer. It was really scary because I didn't want to lose my mom. She talked with me about it every day and that really helped me. I knew that if I ever had any questions about it, I could go to her with them. My mom's cancer wasn't that bad because we detected it at an early stage. I knew that she wasn't going to die, but you can never really be positive.

After my mom had her surgery and radiation treatment, I felt a lot better because we had done something about it. One of the things that helped me the most was God. I prayed to Him every night before bed, which was something that I didn't do a lot. I knew that since I had asked Him for help, He would do the right thing for me. If He had chosen to take my mom away, I knew that He would have a good reason for it.

Mom and I have a very good relationship, and we still talk about her cancer. She doesn't have it any more, but she still has her check-ups to make sure nothing else is growing.

God, my mom and my dad have helped me a lot. I have realized that you should never take things for granted, and you should always make sure that the people you love know that you do love them. I now tell my parents that I love them at least three times a day because I'm never sure if something is going to happen to them. I love them with all my heart and would do anything for them.

31
For My Daddy

by Katie Vaughn (age 15)

Six months ago, my father was diagnosed with multiple myeloma, a very rare, incurable cancer. The battle has been quite a struggle for all of us, but I have learned to stay strong and keep my spirits high. I enjoy researching treatments and studies about the cancer with my father. I ask him many questions about what will happen now and in the future. Knowing my father will not live much longer, I try to make the time we have left as wonderful as possible. I wrote, with much love and concern, a poem about my father and what he goes through every day.

DADDY

So many things that I wish to say,

Before the time in which you must go away.

There's no good place in which I can start,

Because nothing good will come from your last depart.

You gave me life and a reason to live,

But now it's time for me to give.

Why were you stricken with this deadly disease?
I prayed for your life, I begged God please.

I watch you suffer with so much pain,
You're losing your life without any gain.

Before our eyes we watch you fade away,
Because death is the price this cancer makes you
pay.

You've become so weak, you're just not the same,
But it's no one's fault, there's no one to blame.

With all of the wires, tubes and pills that I see,
I realize how bad I'm going to feel when you leave
me.

There's nothing we can do, but to pray and wait,
Because for you to recover it is too late.

God gave you this cancer, knowing there was no
cure,

Knowing that you'd suffer and die for sure.

All those times that I needed you there,

You opened my heart and gave me care.

And from the very moment that you shall die,

Is the exact time my heart will forever cry.

Let's not say good-bye because it's not the end,

Because I know that someday we'll meet again.

And there's one last thing that I've never told you,

I love you, Daddy, and that will always be true.